# Where Are My Car Keys?

Jennylynd James, Ph.D.

# DEDICATION

This book is written in loving memory of my mother, Gloria James, who lived courageously with Alzheimer's disease for many years, until her death in January 2018.

# CONTENTS

# ACKNOWLEDGMENTS

I wish to acknowledge my brother, Lyndon Brent James, and sister, Colette James who shared in this experience as our mother battled with the symptoms of Alzheimer's disease over a period of twelve years. Special thanks to the many friends who dedicated time and attention in the editing and review of this book: Wilma Cayonne, Cynthia Birch, Donna Boyle, Andrea M. William, Fay Sucre, Linus Didier, Leona Thomas, Monica Crane, Aurélie Tauffleib, Deborah Thomas, Lucie Robson, Michael DeGale, Gloria Pelucchia, Felice Gorica, Ann Barrett, Alison Ryan, Paula Crutchley, and Valerie Edwards. Your help and encouragement were greatly appreciated.

# INTRODUCTION

Alzheimer's disease is described as the progressive deterioration of the mind, personality and body, caused by the degeneration of the brain. The disease can begin in late middle age and continue into old age, but what starts the brain's deterioration is yet unknown. Learning about another family's journey can sometimes help in understanding and preparing, if your loved one is diagnosed with Alzheimer's disease.

Everyone is affected by Alzheimer's disease differently, but an emotional rollercoaster is an almost universal journey for caregivers and family members. This book describes our family's voyage, as our mother, Gloria James, 'Mammy', battled Alzheimer's disease over a period of twelve years. It is a collection of stories beginning in 2006 when my siblings and I first acknowledged that our mother's mental and physical states were changing, until her eventual death in January 2018.

One of our concerns was that many elderly parents of our peers in Diamond Vale had also developed Alzheimer's disease, or some other form of dementia. We joked about this, saying there must have been something in the water. We saw a pattern that could not be coincidental, and yet, as far as we knew, nobody was researching this trend.

The cause of this debilitating condition is unknown. Would I develop the disease if my grandmother, mother, uncle and aunt had this condition? Was it truly hereditary? Was it an affliction which plagued people who lived through World War II rations in Trinidad? Was it related to their diet? With so many questions, and no answers, it's difficult not to worry. We don't want to become a statistic.

Jennylynd James

# CHAPTER 1

## IRISH SUPPORT

Beginnings

Armed with a job offer and two large suitcases, we arrived in Dublin Ireland the summer of 2004 to start a new life. My daughter, Tiffany and I had lived in Southern California for almost six years and recently moved to Dublin to seek a new way of life. At the time, I walked with my shoulders back and my nose in the air, as if on a fashion runway. With my long, dark, chemically processed hair, lily white teeth and very dark brown skin, I must have been a curiosity to the other city dwellers. Tiffany at age eight was a happy, carefree child, with olive coloured skin, large round brown eyes, puckered lips, and long, thick brown hair, usually worn in one or two braids. Like any child, she was inquisitive and asked 'Why?' about everything and nothing. I tried to raise her to display the manners and social graces that were becoming of a young lady.

We lived in a modest two-storey home on Dean Swift Road in Glasnevin, Dublin. I purchased this fixer-upper home at the end of 2004 and extensive renovations had been done, breaking down walls to create an open dining room and kitchen area. The former sitting room with a small fireplace was converted into a guest bedroom. Three bedrooms on the second floor were refurbished and painted in bright colours. Old carpets were removed to reveal wooden floors which were sanded, repaired and varnished. The bathrooms on both floors were retiled, with modern sinks and showers installed. The back of the home was extended on the ground level to create a large sunroom looking out onto a 100-foot garden. And the large shed in the backyard was tiled, with electricity installed, providing the ideal storage space. I painted the front of the house yellow and a Georgian style entrance was created with two pillars, a green wooden door, and a brass lion knocker. It was my dream home at the time.

Within two years I decided to quit the job, and started my own business. Once we were all settled in Dublin, my mother wanted to visit us in the summer of 2006. However, my sister Colette, my brother Brent and I had already noticed the uncharacteristic signs of forgetfulness our mother displayed, after being a pillar of strength in our family for decades. The last time we had seen my mother, was in California when she came to visit Tiffany and me. Mammy complained of arthritis in her knees and we had requested wheelchair assistance so she could make her way easily through the large airport terminal in Los Angeles. The vision of a helpless parent at that time stuck with me. Since Mammy enjoyed travelling immensely, we decided that she would have to be accompanied on long distance journeys, involving multiple layovers, from then on. Colette who also enjoyed international travel decided to accompany Mammy with her own two sons, Amiri and Khadir.

My mother, Gloria, was 73 that summer. She was stout and her large frame at five feet seven inches was becoming slightly bent with time. Mammy, as we called her affectionately, had medium length, permed hair which she would set with rollers to curl. Her eyes were large and almond shaped, thoughtfully looking down a long nose with pursed lips. She enjoyed wearing beautiful clothing with matching accessories. My mother lived alone at the family home in Diamond Vale, Diego Martin in Trinidad. When I'd finished high school, my parents got divorced and lived in different towns in Trinidad. My father was experiencing early stages of prostate cancer and the disease seemed to be spreading.

Colette, who lived with her sons in Atlanta, Georgia, couldn't wait to see Ireland. She was like the mythical Amazon women, standing at five feet ten inches tall with big arms and a large frame. Her round face with high cheek bones and slanted almond shaped eyes turned heads. Her sons were aged sixteen and six, and the younger son, Khadir, couldn't sit still. He was always on the move; singing, dancing, and darting here and there. If he fell, he would bounce back up like a rubber ball; there was no stopping him. Khadir had to be monitored closely in airports in case he ran away and got lost. Colette's elder son, Amiri, was over six feet tall, very thin, and quite aware of his good looks. Mammy had travelled on a direct flight from Trinidad to Atlanta and was spending a few months with Colette and her family.

Upon their arrival in Dublin, Colette rented a car at the airport, since I owned a two-seater and couldn't accommodate my clan. Colette shared the guest room with Mammy since it was a large room on the main floor. We didn't want Mammy to have to climb the staircase because of her physical limitations. Amiri was assigned the middle bedroom upstairs, and Tiffany shared her room with Khadir. I had prepared a lengthy itinerary of tourist activities for the family and couldn't wait to show them the sights.

The family complained that my house was too cold, and that Dublin was too cold. I somehow had forgotten to warn them to bring jackets. Even though it was June and temperatures soared to over 30°C in Atlanta where Colette lived, Ireland was seldom hot, with perpetually spring-like temperatures.

'Turn on the heat, yuh cheapskate!' they clamoured.

'No, it's June!' I protested.

'We're never coming back again if you don't turn on the heat!' said Colette.

'That's fine with me,' I said.

Too many family members in a house can be taxing on one's

7

nerves.

Amiri's appearance around Dublin certainly created a stir. He was Mister Friendly and collected an entourage of followers everywhere he went. All the teenagers on Dean Swift Road befriended him immediately. I never knew so many teens lived on my street until Amiri James, or AJ as they called him, arrived. I was known only as AJ's aunt and had no name. Teens visited at various times, day and night, looking for AJ to go into the city centre. Colette and I were worried about his staying out late in a city he didn't know, but AJ was as cool as a cucumber. Sarah, from a few doors down got teased for 'fancying' Amiri. Poor Sarah must have only said hello once, but it was misconstrued as a sign of great affection and that idea stuck.

Ireland Supports Trinidad and Tobago

It was the height of the 2006 FIFA World Cup football tournament in Germany and the team from Trinidad and Tobago had qualified for the first time in its history. The excitement of a Caribbean team representing the region in the finals was enormous. Since we didn't plan to go to Germany to see the matches, we certainly wanted to enjoy the games right there in Dublin.

A week before the Trinidadian team played against Sweden, I had the opportunity to speak for a few seconds on RTÉ radio. I invited Caribbean people and anyone who wanted to support Trinidad to come and watch the match at the Botanic House Pub in Glasnevin the Saturday before my relatives arrived. The turnout was more than I expected, and I made some new friends. Trinidad tied in the match with Sweden and moved on to another match against England.

The Irish were known to support any team that played

against England because of the historical animosity against England, their former conqueror. It so happened that the hosts of my favourite radio show, FM104's Colm and Jim Jim Breakfast Show, decided to throw a party with their sponsors on the evening of June 15th in support of Trinidad and Tobago. I listened to their program religiously every morning and made it a point to call in and win passes for my family and friends to the lavish party. It was sponsored by a brewing company and hosted at The Village Pub on Wexford Street, Dublin.

That evening, I took the whole family down to Wexford Street and witnessed the big party atmosphere, with Brazilian dancers and drummers outside. Did the organisers not realise that Brazil was a slightly different country to Trinidad and Tobago? Oh, never mind, I thought; the atmosphere was fun. We went inside and I enthusiastically introduced myself to the radio hosts, telling them I was from Trinidad. I handed them two music CDs so they could play authentic Trinidadian music at the party. This didn't work, however, and the disc jockeys played miscellaneous 'tropical music'.

Free beer and hors d'oeuvres were provided by the sponsor. With the Trinidad and Tobago flag(s) and a host of decorations, it was almost as good as being back in Trinidad. The hosts conducted competitions and prizes during halftime. That day I wore my hair wide open in the biggest Afro in Dublin. They enjoyed this immensely as I ran up to answer a question and win a DVD player. I think it was because of my mad Afro. Mammy, Colette, the boys and I, sat at the table right in the middle and were highly visible in our Trinidad and Tobago T-shirts. Mammy enjoyed the attention and little Khadir entertained with dances. He was allowed to go wild in the pub, since everyone else was acting wild. It was so encouraging to see all the Irish supporting a country they knew little about.

After halftime, the game resumed.

'Foul! Foul!' we screamed when the English team scored a goal. The referees couldn't hear us. Would Trinidad ever recover? I couldn't breathe with the suspense. It was as if my team had given up. Then the game came to an end.

'No! No! This can't be!' the crowd yelled. 'They cheated. There was a foul. The referee didn't see it!'

The party still went on with music and dancing and people were reluctant to leave, even though it was mid-week with work the next day.

It was the best support Trinidad and Tobago would ever get from total strangers.


Malahide Market

During their first Saturday morning in Dublin, my family decided to accompany me to the Malahide Farmers Market where I had started a new enterprise a few weeks before, selling Caribbean food products. Up until that time, I had never provided details of my business enterprise to the family. Traditionally, selling at markets in the Caribbean was relegated to people considered to be of a low class or uneducated. Trinidad and Tobago was a class conscious society. If one had as many university degrees as me, it was inconceivable to do any manual labour. You were supposed to sit in an office and supervise staff, while making a lot of money. I was worried that the shock of my market stall would kill poor Mammy. I talked about trading at venues, plans for wholesale operations, promoting Caribbean food, being the first in Ireland to run this kind of business, being a pioneer; everything but selling at farmers markets.

As I prepared cooked snacks for the market, my sister said,

'Let me help. Let me help.'

But as I cooked, she kept scolding me.

'That's not the way to make aloo pie. Saheenas don't look like that. Why are you only using one baking tray for coconut drops? Shouldn't you buy some more baking trays?'

By the time we got to pie number 30, she was tired, said I had great patience, and sat down to relax. She vowed never to do that type of work.

I had hired Paul, a jovial young man from Jamaica, a few weeks before to help me at the markets. He had the gift of the gab, which was a much-needed skill to make money. He was very good at charming the ladies and speaking with the lads to make sales. Paul met us near the Malahide Marina and we set up the tent, put up decorative flags and set out the tables and products for sale. Setting up took longer than usual, since my whole family had followed me in the rental car and everyone wanted to help, even Mammy. I had to beg them to take a walk around and look at the other vendors who sold delicious cakes, jams, and other goodies.

'Leave Paul to set up please,' I urged them.

My mother shook her head in disapproval and disgust. 'So much education. So much education. I can't believe this. I sent her to university and this is what she's doing? Shameful.'

Mammy lamented to my sister repeatedly and they both shook their heads while I remained optimistic for a profitable day at the market. My nephew wanted to try selling when everything was set up, and started singing a Caribbean folk song as an elderly couple approached the tent. However, he managed to frighten away these potential customers. After observing his antics, I decided it was enough. While Paul worked at our booth, I took the family for a drive up the coast to visit the seaside town of Howth. Anything was better than frightening away customers! At the end of the work day I returned to pack up with Paul and collect the proceeds. Paul managed to cover the expenses of the rent and his wages with very little to spare. I asked several market vendors if I should be hiring more helpers to sell my products.

'Nobody would sell as well as you,' they said. 'Don't waste your money.'

Travel Adventures

The following week, I kept the family very busy with sight seeing trips. We did the Hop On - Hop Off bus tour of Dublin and a day trip to Wicklow County to see the Powers Court Waterfalls and Glendalough. I drove along the coast stopping at the beaches in Dalkey, Bray and other Dublin and Wicklow towns. Mammy seemed excited by all the new sites. However, she kept mixing up the names of places and counties. It was a lot for her to digest. We also took a day trip to the National Aquatic Centre, where we tried out all the slides and tubes and other attractions.

I observed small changes in my mother's behaviour when I took her out one day for a drive and to have tea. We visited Phoenix Park, the largest park in Dublin and I showed her some of the beautiful gardens, the cricket pitch and deer roaming freely in some areas. We then went to the tea rooms at the Visitor Centre. My mother mumbled incessantly about nothing and looked visibly uncomfortable. I tried to put her at ease, but it didn't work. In the past, she would thoroughly have enjoyed the trip because she used to love sightseeing and going out to tea. She walked slowly and tentatively, and one knee was bent in slightly to meet the other. Little did I know, that her constant mumbling and feeling uncomfortable, were just the start of a downward spiral leading to Alzheimer's.

Barbecue

The following Saturday I threw a barbecue party to celebrate summer and introduce the family to my friends and favourite neighbours. I invited many Dublin friends: the Hennessys, the Callallys, and a new Trinidadian family I met quite by accident. Everything was fine except that the barbecue grill was still in its original box! I started assembling the grill during the party and it never quite stood up correctly. Those little kettle grills were not always reliable and I didn't know how to assemble it. I called on one of the guests for assistance so we could get the meat over the charcoals, but as a time saving measure, baked everything in the oven. The meat was cooked by the time the grill was assembled.

The party was great fun for the children who bounced on Tiffany's huge trampoline for hours. Most of the guests sat in the sun room at the back of the house and a few under the umbrella on the back patio in the garden. The sunroom also served as the TV room. Since the World Cup matches were still taking place, we let the TV run during the party so those consumed by World Cup Fever could watch.

'Shaka Hislop of Pearl Parkway, Diamond Vale, Diego Martin!' My mother screamed at the television as advertising came on air.

Shaka Hislop, the goal keeper of the Trinidad and Tobago World Cup football team, was a former neighbour who grew up on the same street where I was raised in Trinidad - Pearl Parkway, Diamond Vale, Diego Martin. His family was always involved in sports and we felt proud to know he was representing our country.

'Why is your mother talking to the television,' asked a good friend.

'She always does that. No big deal,' I replied. The concern was whether she thought the announcer was talking back to her. Mammy lived alone at her home in Trinidad and enjoyed watching a US Game Show Network all day and night. Colette remembered seeing my mother shout answers at the television and even ask her little dog to answer the questions the show participants couldn't answer. This was one of her favourite pastimes. We took her behaviour lightly at that time and mistakenly thought it may have been brought on by loneliness.

Journey Home

After a few days, the family returned to Atlanta. Colette protested about having to keep them all together as a unit.

'I have to be the guide dog for all of them!' she joked.

One strategy to keep the group together was to push my mother along in a wheelchair. She was unable to walk quickly and became tired easily. This was the sensible option. In addition, if Mammy was seated in a wheelchair, she would be less likely to wander off unnoticed.

The stories I heard about their adventures in the airport made me chuckle.

Khadir ran around the food hall, almost getting lost, Amiri continued to chase after girls who admired his height, and Mammy attempted to go in search of the washroom on her own in the departure lounge and had to be brought back to safety. Great patience was required. I also heard that the stack of passports was accidentally forgotten on a table in the Dublin Airport food court. Colette had to retrace her steps to find them before going through security.

She would never volunteer for such a mission again.

## CHAPTER 2

## HOME FOR THE HOLIDAYS

Happy Holidays 2007

Tiffany and I were leaving Ireland to spend Christmas in Trinidad and we couldn't wait. Christmas in Trinidad was one of my favourite holidays. It meant many days of eating delicious food, and listening to exciting Christmas music like Parang, the vibrant folk music sung in Spanish. Parang music was brought to Trinidad and Tobago by Spanish speaking Venezuelan and Colombian migrants. It was tradition in the past for Parang singers and musicians to visit homes of family and friends at night, waking them up and performing for food and drinks. A 'Trini' Christmas meant eating ham, pastels (corn meal dish filled with meat), black fruit cake (usually made with rum), souse (fresh pickled pigs' feet), and drinking sorrel (red drink made from a hibiscus type flower), ginger beer and Peardrax (a carbonated drink). I would seldom get this food while living outside of Trinidad and I was already sweetening my chops from a distance with the mere thought of the feast to come.

We left Dublin and flew to Heathrow Airport in the UK. While waiting in the Heathrow departure lounge, my accent immediately changed from pseudo-Irish to a Trinidadian accent. All I had to do was listen to the Trinis around me, and bingo, I became one.

'Mommy, why are you speaking like that?' asked Tiffany.

'Ah practicing for when ah reach mih Island gyurl!' I explained.

The ten-hour flight was shear torture, to say the least. How much cheap airline food could one possibly stomach? Frequent announcements made it difficult to get a nap, so I tossed and turned or walked the aisles a few times. As we were landing in Piarco Airport in Trinidad, passengers celebrated the touchdown with loud applause in true Trinidadian style. I wondered if we were the only nationals to applaud when we got back to our home of birth. Everybody had the same conversations of visiting family, exchanging gifts and eating and drinking.

'Ah want ah piece ah pork for mih Christmas!' The Soca Parang parties were beckoning.

When we arrived, my mother had come to the airport to meet us. She was going to be 75 in a few days and was a bit forgetful. However she was still able to drive and truly enjoyed it. Driving was a significant part of her freedom. She drove fast, and everyone had to look out when Mammy was on the road.

'Yuh see how dat one try to give mih a bad drive? What de hell wrong wid he?' she would say.

Mammy blew the car horn frequently, so trouble makers would know she owned the road! When we stopped at a traffic light at the junction of Diego Martin Highway and St Lucian Road, the light turned green suddenly. The driver behind us who was obviously in a hurry to eat his Christmas meal blew his horn. That certainly brought out the wrath of Gloria James.

'Pass over mih! See if yuh could drive over mih!' she screamed, motioning with her index finger to the driver.

Tiffany giggled in the back seat and I was too distressed from the lengthy travel to get into a fight with a passing car. As we took off, the car behind quickly over took us with the driver glaring at the old woman who thought the road belonged to her. I was happy to get to the house in one piece and promised to get into the driver's seat for the rest of the trip in order to preserve my sanity.

We arrived at my childhood home on Pearl Parkway, Diamond Vale, Diego Martin. Everything looked well maintained since my mother had done renovations on the front of the house. The only difference this time was that the house had been painted a shocking pink! It was a cross between peach and loud fuchsia, and not easy to understand.

'How yuh like de house? De painter was really good,' she said.

'Well, it certainly looks different,' I said, trying to control my shock.

What was she thinking? But by then her brain was truly playing tricks on her. I was assigned the guest room with an en suite bathroom at the back of the house since my partner Sean was coming from Ireland on vacation just after Christmas. Tiffany got the middle bedroom and my childhood bedroom which had two twin sized beds, was reserved for my sister Colette and her son, Khadir who were flying in from the United States the following day.

'La La La … Drink a rum … La La La!' sang Mammy.

We were awoken by loud music from a noisy radio at 6:30 am. My mother woke up early and walked around, singing and making breakfast.

'Why? Why?' I wanted to ask. 'Did we really have to wake up so early?'

'All yuh wake up for breakfast,' Mammy called from the kitchen.

The rooster on Gopaul Avenue crowed, the birds in the garden chirped and every neighbour's dog barked in the morning.

A kiskadee, the colourful and noisy tropical bird, was very persistent in his calls that morning. 'Kiss ka dee ... Kiss ka dee ...'

The cacophony of sound was punctuated by the blowing horn of the fish monger as he called out, 'Carete, Cavali and Shark!'

I must have forgotten what it was like in Diamond Vale in the morning. Everything happened early. Trinidadians were early risers and life started at 4:30 am for some. There was no sleeping late like in other cultures.

We rose early, enjoyed our breakfast, and then prepared to return to the airport to collect Colette and Khadir. With a full house, we had more noise and confusion.

'Let's buy roti! No let's buy Chinese food! No let's buy fried chicken!'

Everything tasted better in Trinidad. It must have been the seasoning and the sun ripened fruits and vegetables. Even a cucumber had a strong and delicious flavour compared to cucumbers grown in other climates.

'But we shouldn't be eating out. We should focus on the Christmas menu,' I protested.

My mother said she had already bought food for Christmas. However, when we checked the refrigerator and cupboards, it was obviously supplies for only one person and not for the four invaders who arrived from abroad. We went to the supermarket on Diamond Boulevard. It was still affectionately called the Co-op, the original supermarket formed as a cooperative way back in the 1970s. I still remembered sitting through the grand opening speeches on hard metal chairs in the car park, and the delicious cheese puffs and beef pies served to attendees on the day. A child only focuses on the important details. The Diego Martin Consumers Cooperative Society Limited, the Co-op had been bought out by a supermarket chain but had the same face as it did so many decades before.

'My daughters are visiting from AWAY,' said Mammy to anyone who would listen to her in the supermarket.

'You don't have to tell everyone,' I protested. 'That will just alert the bandits!'

Our home had been burgled several times in the 1980's and it was a period when everyone installed metal burglar proof gratings on windows, doors, and other entrances. The brisk business of artistic looking, patterned iron cages changed the faces of houses in our beloved Diamond Vale.

It was surprising how well-mannered Trinidadians could be. Everyone greeted the other saying 'Good morning'. I felt a tinge of guilt if I ignored anyone. After living outside the country in large cities where people seldom greeted each other, it was a rare treat to observe the human interaction in Trinidad. I was aghast at the food prices that seemed extra high, even for locally grown vegetables. At the check-out someone actually packed my bags for me and brought the bags out to the car. That too was a rare treat, long discontinued in so-called developed countries.

Colette and I whipped up a Christmas menu and thought back fondly on the old Christmas days. The anticipation of Christmas in the old days was infectious. Weeks of cleaning and tumbling up the house, last minute painting, polishing floors and shining furniture, were part of the Christmas frenzy.

'Don't walk on the floors I've just polished. Stay out of the living room. We can't put up a Christmas tree in a dirty house! That area is for when company comes!' we would say in the good old days.

Many beautiful things were designated to the mysterious 'company' that was supposed to visit. This was no fun for a child. The cleaning frenzy was followed by a cooking frenzy. I was not sure when gift buying fit in. Having lived in other countries, the focus seemed to be more on shopping and buying gifts. Boiling of salty, preserved European ham used to be a very important activity. The ham came tarred and dried from somewhere far away. Apples and grapes were considered exotic fruits and we only got them once a year from Ibrahim Wholesalers in Port-of-Spain. Black fruit cake was baked a week in advance and my mother prepared fresh bread and sweet bread on Christmas Eve. A fresh pork leg and the ham leg dressed with cloves and pineapple slices went into the oven on Christmas Eve, and the Christmas turkey went into the oven after returning from midnight mass, so it could bake for hours while we slept.

That year, we wondered if we should go to midnight mass at St Michael's and All Angels Anglican Church on the Boulevard. Our childhood tradition on Christmas Eve was to go to midnight mass when we would invariably nod through the lengthy service. Then we'd visit our friends, the O'Neills on Sapphire Drive, to get a taste of their pastels, ham, and black fruit cake. It was as if nobody slept on Christmas Eve in anticipation of the big day to follow. As children, we kept one eye open, hoping to get a glimpse of Santa Claus, who would mysteriously leave gifts on our bed. Our father, Kenneth, who usually partied with his buddies singing from house to house, would bring friends to our house for drinks in the wee hours of the morning; maybe 2:00 am. They would all be inebriated by that time, pretending to sing Parang songs. We would bring out food and drinks for the group, as was our tradition, and hope that they'd move on to another house swiftly so we could get some sleep. I remembered my mother warning Daddy to come home after the next house and not go any further with 'the boys'. He was filled with drinks and she wanted him home and in good shape for the big Christmas breakfast, and the even bigger Christmas lunch later in the day.

Alas, as adults returning from foreign countries, we had no such feelings of anticipation and excitement for Christmas. We were not waiting for Santa Claus, and a fairly clean house was good enough. Christmas Eve, we didn't go to midnight mass and relaxed just trying to recover from jet lag. Christmas morning however, we were awoken by the radio playing loud celebration music again.

'Neighbah, La La La is Christmas ... Neighbah, La La La is Christmas.'

Mammy was awake and the radio was making a racket as usual. We had no choice but to wake up. It was time to exchange gifts before our sumptuous breakfast feast. Khadir, being the youngest, received more toys than he could ever imagine. He was as happy as could be. Tiffany also received toys and clothes. She was in between childhood and teenage years, a strange time for gift giving, since she felt too old for toys.

Christmas Day was quiet, and from childhood, it always seemed like an anti-climax to the weeks of preparation. If only we could experience the same feeling of anticipation throughout the day. We called friends and planned ahead for parties for the rest of the holidays. In the evening we visited the Hackshaws on the Boulevard, to taste their Christmas ham and cake. Then we visited the Pierres for some Christmas cheer. Christmas day was open house for many families in the neighbourhood. The Adams family on Manning Street in Diego Martin usually hosted a family gathering on Boxing Day, complete with Parang music, food and drink. This was their family tradition for decades, and whenever we happened to return to Trinidad on holidays, we jumped into their family reunion as if we'd never left. The good thing about these gatherings was that they were intergenerational. My mother got dressed up for the occasion, and Colette, Tiffany Khadir and I were ready too. We danced, sang, ate and drank and when the Parang group came, we danced again. It was the same group that would visit our house every year when we threw a party for our mother's birthday on December 29th; Los Paranderos en Coches (The Parang singers in cars). Sauntering home after Boxing Day celebrations, I prepared for my partner, Sean who was arriving from Ireland the next day for his first visit to Trinidad and Tobago.

The Irishman Comes to Trinidad

Feeling overstuffed from the Christmas menu and leftovers, we were looking forward to feasting on an Asian style menu for my mother's upcoming birthday party. We had two days to relax the stomachs before the next feast.

'After eating so much food, I think ah need a purge!' I said.

In the good old days, we would drink senna pods tea or Milk of Magnesia to flush out the stomach after over eating. I never did get a purge, but continued feasting to enjoy the holidays thoroughly.

Sean was flying from Dublin on St Stephen's Day and we were to have 10 days in Trinidad and Tobago for fun and adventure. He had never been to Trinidad and I welcomed the opportunity to show him the sights. We were also celebrating my mother's 75th birthday, so it was a grand family occasion.

Sean managed to get a flight to Scarborough, Tobago from London, and then he flew to Port-of-Spain on a one-way ticket. The plan was for us to return to Tobago after the New Year for a visit before he returned to Ireland.

My mother's house had no air-conditioning and the mosquitoes loved fresh blood, so he was in for a treat; a baptism of fire. I imagined he'd be completely exhausted from over ten hours of commuting and would want to go directly to bed. When Colette and I met him at the airport that night, Sean was bouncing off the walls and full of energy.

'I want to go to the beach,' said Sean as soon as he entered the car.

'And Happy Christmas to you too… It's too late Sean. Nobody's in the water at this time,' I said. 'In any case, the best beaches are on the north coast and they're too far from here!'

'No way,' he said. 'I've come all the way from Ireland. I have to get a bath in the sea. It's too hot. I need a swim.'

We could not convince him that it was night and we were not physically close to any beaches at the airport, even though we were on an island. Sean was an avid swimmer. He lived near the coast and would swim everyday if he had the opportunity. There was no stopping him. We decided to take him for a dip at Dean's Bay, Carenage, about forty minutes away. This was against our better judgement, since we believed people in our circles would never go there, and certainly not at night. It could have been dangerous. All the locals we had spoken with, warned us repeatedly about staying away from lonely places at night, because it was so dangerous!

We drove along the narrow road leading down to Carenage. Passing through Point Cumana, Sean observed the little shops and the loud music emanating from bars with delight!

'Oh we should stop there,' he exclaimed.

'Not at all,' I said. 'We don't go to rum shops! Are you crazy?'

'Well, I would go to a rum shop' he said. It was the dream of every tourist to boldly go where we had not gone before. As we turned the bend approaching Dean's Bay, we looked at the dark and deserted area. There was not much of a beach, just a narrow strip of sand with small rocks and pebbles. A handful of brave souls were in the water and three cars were parked nearby. A few people were relaxing and drinking near their cars.

'You see, people are liming near the water, Sean, but they're not in it,' said Colette.

'Liming? What's liming?' asked Sean.

'That's when you sit and chat with friends. Sometimes people lime and hangout, eating food and also with a few drinks,' she explained.

'Well I'm going in,' he repeated. 'It's way too hot.'

If only he knew that the night time temperature was at least five degrees cooler than midday. He would melt when he experienced reality the next day. Sean had a habit of stripping and changing right in front of anyone at his local beach in Ireland. I had to convince him to find a changing room before he started undressing at Dean's Bay. Luckily there was an old wooden building with changing rooms next to a tiny police station, and they were still open. Sean ran in and swiftly returned, wearing his new tropical swimming trunks. He prepared well for his Caribbean vacation.

He threw his clothes and bag into the back seat of the car and before we could even ask a question, he ran towards the water. He went diving head first, while Colette and I said a prayer for his safety from the Boogeyman who lived in the ocean at night. We never dared enter the water at night. Dean's Bay with its muddy sea floor, full of silt dumped by rivers during the rainy season was not enticing to us. Sean surfaced and then went under again. We had to stop our useless fretting and let the man enjoy his first dip in a Trinidadian sea.

'Woohoo! That water's nice! Oh it's fabulous!' Sean yelled. He emerged from the dark shore as we looked nervously left and right for possible bandits who might try to rob us of Mammy's little old car and the small change in our handbags.

'Oh no, the changing room's closed. I'll have to change right here!' he said, and without hesitation, Sean dropped his swimming trunks and dried himself quickly with a towel from one of his bags. He had no problem with modesty and we hoped those in the other cars were not seeing through the faint night lights.  Sean changed into some summer gear, shorts and a t-shirt. 'Where to next?' he asked fully refreshed and ready for exploration.

'Well, I'll stop to buy roti at Don's Roti Shop in Petit Valley,' I said, driving away from Dean's Bay rapidly. The discomfort of looking for potential thieves had been too much for us. The area was probably safe, but we had heard too many stories about robberies and attacks in quiet areas, and we did not want to take any chances.

As we neared Don's Roti shop and bar on St Lucien Road, I asked Sean what type of roti he'd like to get: chicken, beef or goat. He had never tasted goat roti even though I'd prepared curry for him in the past, so he was quite excited by the prospect of consuming local food.

'I'll pop in and place the order and Colette can stay with the car to find parking,' I said.

Sean, of course wanted to come out to see what a roti shop looked like. The building was a simple concrete structure and a counter top with burglar proof gratings through which patrons placed their orders. As we walked in, everyone turned to stare at Sean and me. Their eyes seemed to ask, who was the pale white man in a Hawaiian t-shirt, short pants and flip flops, and what was he doing in their roti shop. Trinidadians usually stared long and hard at each other. It was normal to examine a person from head to toe and back up before removing the gaze. I tried to sink into the ground as Sean and I walked in, but it wasn't possible since the place was too small to hide.

I placed an order for our rotis and said we would take them home to eat.

'Oh no,' said Sean. I want to eat right here!'

'No Sean, no! This is like a rum shop. People in our circles would never sit and drink here. We go to more fancy pubs,' I explained.

'Oh you're so snobbish. I see nothing wrong with the place. I want a beer,' he said.

I realised then and there, I was going to have a challenging time keeping an eye on Sean in Trinidad and keeping him safe.

Before I could say any more, he ordered drinks and sat down at the front near the roadway. My sister who was waiting in the car had no choice but to join us. Waiting for our roti order took a long time, so Sean had enough time to observe John Public, and they him.

'We never sit here to eat Sean,' Colette confirmed. 'Our friends don't come here. We just buy the roti and leave.'

'I've told him that already,' I said. 'This man will raise my blood pressure during his trip!'

Just as I complained, a drunken man fell to the floor near the table next to us. He was holding a drink which also fell with him. The man wore dark sunglasses, a t-shirt and jeans and a cap turned backwards on his head. He had been drinking alone and many people waiting for their rotis or standing at the bar next door turned to see what the commotion was about.

'Yes!' screamed Sean. 'I feel like I'm in Ireland. I feel at home! Let's drink to dat!'

We raised our bottles to the drunk. When we got our roti, Colette and I ate nervously, as we looked around at the clientele and passing cars. Again, stories about random shootings and robberies in the Diego Martin and Petit Valley areas had us on edge and we just could not relax as we sat at the corner of a major thoroughfare.

Eventually we finished food and drinks and hastily ushered our visitor out to the car. My mother was waiting for us when we arrived home.

'You got back late! Why are you so late?' she asked.

By then it was 10:00 pm and she had no hesitation in greeting her new house guest while staring at him and asking a million questions. Sean liked all the attention he was getting. He felt like a million dollars until a mosquito bit his leg. We were sharing the guest bedroom at the back of the house and it was the most private bedroom in our family home.

Poor Sean provided free dinner for all the mosquitoes in the guest bedroom that night. Even though we were equipped with citronella oil, bug spray and a bug mat, the highly skilled mosquitoes found their way to his skin. By morning, he had several red bumps on his arms and legs. He refused to cover up at night because it was too hot to sleep.

'Lindy how could you bring me to a place with no air-conditioning?' he asked.

'When in Rome do as the Romans do,' I said. 'Houses seldom have air-conditioning in the tropics. We are saving the planet and you can probably get used to the heat.'

However, I doubted this was possible in a short stay of just one week.

'Seany! Seany!' my mother was calling around 6:30 am next morning. We were both in a deep slumber finally, after wrestling with the heat, insect bites, and constant night noises of singing frogs and crickets.

'Oh, I forgot to mention, everything starts early in Trinidad. My mother wakes up at the crack of dawn to prepare breakfast,' I said.

He just turned and put the pillow over his head. It was very difficult explaining our early morning customs to a visitor. He just couldn't understand, because he was on vacation.

'What's all that racket about? Why are the birds chirping so loudly?' asked Sean.

'Oh that's the resident kiskadee. He has to greet everyone at least a hundred times. Work starts early at many businesses because the midday sun is so hot,' I said.

We could hear the outdoor labourers on the street in front of the houses as they called out to each other while cutting grass. They always started early and by mid-morning they could be seen relaxing. By lunch time, they would be gone. The locals joked about this as a half day's work for a full day's wage.

'Seany, Seany,' called Mammy again.

'I guess we can't disappoint her,' I said. 'She's prepared breakfast for you. We can plan our strategy of places to visit since we're up early anyway.'

Sean reluctantly dragged himself off the bed and into the shower. It would be the first of many showers for the day since one could readily sit still and sweat all day.

'I need to get to a beach,' he said, reaffirming that he was on a Caribbean island. He vowed to get to a beach every single day. Luckily I had asked my cousin, Richard to rent us a car from his 'fleet' for a few days when Sean was in town. It was one way for us to be totally independent on our visit. Richy was to bring the car for us that morning. My cousin was described as the family's entrepreneur, the one to contact for anything under the sun. If Richy couldn't do it, nobody could. He ran several businesses, and car sales and rentals was just one of them. At the time he was importing and re-selling foreign, used Japanese cars. He brought us a beautiful, medium-sized caramel coloured car. It still had the new car smell and was equipped with air-conditioning, which was a God-send in the 30-degree plus temperatures.

'Take good care of my car folks,' he said. 'I still have to sell it!'

'No problem,' I said. 'We'll just go around town and to a few beaches. That's all!'

After breakfast we got dressed and arranged to meet my friend Lucia and her son to visit the north coast of Trinidad. Tiffany was ready early, and with a car full of sightseers, we made our way up the north coast to hop from beach to beach. It had been a few years since I saw the beaches on the north coast and was determined to follow the road all the way to the end. The first stop was at the look out point just before Maracas Beach. This was a place where one could park and take in the scenery. Two or three vendors sold from large booths filled with traditional sweets, snack foods, and preserves. The look out point provided the most spectacular views of the untouched northern coastline. Green peninsulas could be seen jutting out into the deep blue sea. We took many photos and dodged the man with the guitar who felt it was his duty to terrorize every sight-seer with a song for a few dollars.

'Sorry, we're not interested. Just want to look at the view.'

The musician/folk singer was persistent, especially when he spotted Sean, the tourist. I stocked up on local treats like sugar cake, tooloom, tamarind balls, pepper mango, bene balls, shaddock, peanut brittle, pomecythere chow, and pineapple chow. My order may have been one of the largest the vendor had seen that day. As we drove away along the coast road, I wondered if we would be able to eat all those snack foods. I bought them for sentimental reasons and this was always the dilemma. I could never get these items in Ireland, so I felt compelled to buy them.

Our goal was to drive along the Coast Road to where it ended at Blanchiseusse, a village located about midway along the north coast of Trinidad. We stopped at each beach along the way, took a few photos and then continued on the course: Maracas, Tyrico Bay, Las Cuevas Beach, and others along the popular north coast. At Blanchisseuse, the water was rough that day and we didn't dare go in. Walking around the village, Sean spotted a rum shop and we all went in to see what they had on sale. We ordered soft drinks and Sean's eye caught a poster for a drink called Correia's Hard Wine. The poster showed a beautiful young woman in a swim suit and explained that Hard Wine consisted of ingredients that promoted stamina & power. The alcoholic drink was described as a blend of fruit wine with herbal extracts, and a distinctive taste. Sean could not resist

ordering a glass of hard wine for the adventure. It was one
of the highlights of his trip to the north coast.


75th Birthday and Old Year's Night

Mammy's 75th birthday party took place next day on
December 29th at a restaurant on Ariapita Avenue. The
restaurant we chose was popular for its Asian fusion food
and my brother contacted his event planner to arrange all
the details for the party. The event planner booked the
restaurant, chose the menu, and sent out invitations. She also
reserved a Parang band that was supposed to come later in
the evening to sing Christmas songs and perform music for
dancing.  All we had to do was get my mother ready for the
occasion and participate in the program. I had bought a gold
dress for Mammy in Ireland, and some matching costume
jewellery. With mild Alzheimer's disease symptoms she had
become a little stubborn at times. We got many questions
and resistance.

'Where am I going?' asked Mammy. 'I'm not wearing that! I
said I'm not wearing that!'

'It's your birthday party. Many of your friends will be
coming,' I said.

Two hours later, she asked me the same question. 'Where
am I going? Which restaurant is it? Who's coming?'

We had been through the arrangements a few times, but it
was no use. Her short term memory was gone.

'Is Seany coming too?' she asked suddenly.

'Yes he is, and he'll dance with you at the party,' I said.

She liked the sound of that and was delighted to be dancing

with Sean from Ireland. I helped my mother get dressed, brushed her hair and put on minimal makeup. Doing her hair and nails were a bit challenging because she wouldn't sit still, and I had to get dressed too.

We arrived half an hour early to the venue to be sure everything was in place. We walked to the second floor of the restaurant designated for special events, in time to observe the staff running around in a frenzy, as they set up the room at the last minute. Luckily the event planner was available to work with them. I expected everything to be ready hours in advance. Colette, Khadir, Sean, Tiffany, Mammy and I sat at a table and waited patiently for the room to be readied and the guests to arrive. In true 'Trini fashion', i.e. late, people trickled in slowly and long after the starting time.

'What place is this?' Mammy asked. 'Why are we here again?'

We had a few appetisers at each table and I walked around greeting people I hadn't seen in a long time. Tiffany and Khadir entertained their Granny with stories. Our family sat at the head table which was decorated with candles and a big banner hanging from the wall that showed my mother's photo and the words Happy 75th Birthday. Seats were assigned at the tables, with some of my mother's closest friends sitting with us at the head table. Her childhood friend, Gloria, who was also an ordained Anglican priest, joined us at the head table to start the event with a prayer. When most of the guests arrived, we started a short program of speeches and songs. Dinner was a delicious buffet of Christmas favourites and Oriental dishes: ham, turkey, pastels, shrimp chow mein, char su pork, fried rice, and other dishes. The smells emanating from the buffet table made us extra hungry as we piled food on our plates. It was a grand feast and everyone seemed happy.

Then the house DJ started playing Trinidadian Christmas music like Soca Parang, Parang, and Jazzy Carols, and Mammy took to the dance floor with friends. She loved dance music and her bent knee didn't stop her from doing a little two step. During the desert course, Khadir sang the happy birthday song and Tiffany also sang. My mother's niece, Gemma who arrived later than everyone else, decided to give a speech. She told everyone she was 'waiting for passage' to come into town for the party, which was why she was late.

My mother, who couldn't remember Gemma replied, 'Who is she? And who invited her to my party anyway?'

Luckily only the people at the head table heard this remark. Eyes rolled and Tiffany and Khadir snickered uncontrollably. It would have been quite embarrassing for poor Gemma if she'd heard. The party continued to swing when the Parang band arrived singing their melodious Spanish songs to celebrate the festive Christmas Season.

'Rio Manzanare dejame pasar…'

Mammy announced that she had to dance. 'I have to dance with Seany who came all the way from Ireland just for my birthday party!'

He laughed heartily and agreed to dance with her. He was also a bit drunk by that time and enjoyed all her nonsensical comments. Mammy danced so much at her party and we secretly wondered if she would remember anything the following day. Such was the plight of the birthday girl with Alzheimer's disease.

More Parties

The dust settled and the very next day we were out

sightseeing and planning for more events. On Old Year's Night, we joined the Adams family for their celebration at Edwin's home in Petit Valley. All children, parents and grandparents, joined in the fun to ring in the New Year. Many generations could be seen at the party and it was one good reason to attend. Mammy sat with Mrs. Adams and her friends and smiled sweetly making conversation.

Colette and I marvelled at how well Mammy fit in, considering she didn't recognise anybody.

'Do those people realise Mammy doesn't know who they are? She's putting on a good show,' said Colette.

Since she acted normal in a party setting nobody knew her mental state. The music was too loud for serious conversion anyway, so she was fine.

We sent Tiffany to socialize with the teenagers, and Khadir ran wild with many small children on site. We hoped he wouldn't get into too much mischief, but he was always into mischief. Colette, Sean and I mingled with the middle-aged parents talking about our good old days and all the parties we attended in our youth. The family hosted the backyard party around a beautiful swimming pool. It was an occasion for us to celebrate the wealth of our Trini friends, ringing in the New Year. I felt Sean was impressed with the crowd and the abundance around him and he got merry and slightly drunk.

Soka in Moka

A new year had started and new Soca songs filled the airwaves. It was New Year's Day 2008 and the short Carnival season in Trinidad and Tobago beckoned with the Carnival parade scheduled for February 19th and 20th,

Carnival nation had to try as best as possible to squeeze in parties and events into a mere six-week period. For this reason, Soka in Moka, one of the most popular College Alumni All Inclusive fetes, was planned for January 1st. All Trini Expats visiting for Christmas were as pleased as punch to get a jump-up and wine before returning to our respective cold and dreary climates. I was happy to also have Sean sample a little taste of Trinidad Carnival.

We purchased our party tickets well in advance, got dressed by early afternoon and made our way over Morne Coco Road to Maraval Road leading to Moka. Morne Coco Road was narrow and winding, with small houses and some shacks precariously perched on the sides of steep hills. Sean observed the scenery and was visibly shaken when we turned a bend near a precipice. His comfort level settled when we eventually arrived on flat land at Maraval Road. This road was also narrower than he was used to, with racing traffic heading in both directions. As we entered the Moka district, houses became larger and larger. Sean's eyes opened wide. He couldn't believe the wealth in front of him. Ostentatious homes with neatly manicured gardens could be seen on both sides of the route. There was new construction of town houses and enormous wrought iron gates with intricate designs of all patterns.

'Why are these houses so big?' he asked. 'It's not fair to the people who don't have money. I can't believe these people could have such big houses and there are other people barely living on the poverty line. It just seems unfair to me.'

Colette and I looked at each other in amusement and we let him rant for a while.

We presented our tickets and walked in to inspect the food pavilions. There was Creole food, Chinese food, Indian food, and every other imaginable American style meal too. My partner was fascinated by all the drinks Pavilions: rum, beer, cocktails, whiskey and more.

'And everyone could drink and go back for more?' asked Sean. 'How is this possible for one price?'

'Well,' I said. 'It's going to be a drinker's paradise!'

As the night went on, more and more people arrived and the music rang out from large speakers on one side of the grounds then a live performance began on another side. People ate and danced like there was no tomorrow. Then they drank and danced. When the sun went down, more people arrived and the merriment continued … eat and dance, drink and dance, then eat again. As a non-drinker, I was determined to make the most of all the food being served to get my money's worth! Sean paced himself with the drinks, but he was enjoying the lime.

We entered one of the drinks pavilions and a few white Trinidadians were dancing and partying over there. Sean approached a man with dark hair and asked him if he was Irish.

'No man, Ah from right here,' said the man.

'Are you sure?' asked Sean, not convinced the man was telling the truth.

Up to that time, Sean had mainly seen Trinidadians of various colours and races. He had not seen his own kind and may have been somewhat relieved and ready to bond. I had to tell him that not every white person was Irish. As Sean got a little tipsy, he spied a redheaded woman dancing in the crowd and of course had to approach her since she may have looked Irish too.

'Hello, you must be Irish,' he said with certainty.

'No, I'm British actually,' said the woman.

'So what are you doing here?' asked Sean.

'Well, my best friend is from Trinidad and I'm here for a visit,' she responded.

'That's just like you being here Sean,' I reminded him, and had to pull him away to another area so he would not continue to bother 'Irish-looking' people. His behaviour was amusing.

At 11:00 pm sharp, the loud music wound down and then a small steelband with pans around the neck started playing 'oldie goldies'. People danced around the small band as the musicians strategically started moving towards the gates.

'I don't understand how they could still be sober,' said Sean. 'If this were in Ireland, people would be drunk on the floor. The bar was giving away the alcohol! Irish people would drink until there was nothing left!'

It was his turn to be amused. Trinidadians didn't drink the bar dry.

Trip to Tobago

Seany bid my mother farewell two days later when we travelled by ferry to Tobago.

'I'll miss you Seany,' she said, and gave him a big hug.

He enjoyed being my mother's favourite for the day and told her that he'd return again just to see her another time.

Sean seemed to settle mentally when we flew to Tobago for a few days and stayed in a hotel by the sea. He could have the comfort of an air-conditioned room that was not available at my mother's house, and the mosquitoes ignored him. His skin was already a rare polka dot pattern after a week in Diego Martin. In Tobago, the tourist island of Trinidad and Tobago, Sean saw many German tourists and others from Europe. He felt easier around his own kind.

We rented a car and travelled around the island, beach-hopping and eating, then visited my father's cousin, Phyllis in St Cecelia. She and her husband were retired and frequently hosted lavish parties at their home inviting other retired friends. My father was also on vacation in Tobago at Phyllis' home that week, and so we had the opportunity to hang out with him. Everyone ate, drank and drank some more.

When we returned to the hotel, my heart was heavy, because I was leaving my sweetheart all alone in Tobago for two days, returning to Trinidad to catch my flight back to Ireland. I felt anxious about leaving Sean, a 50 year old grown man, as if he was my absent-minded child.

'Let me pay the bill. The price will go up if they hear your accent. Take the taxi over there to get back to Store Bay. Stay out of trouble. Don't trust anyone. Try not to get robbed. Put your wallet in your front pocket, not the back pocket. Ask the taxi not to take you on the scenic route.'

I spouted endless instructions before taking ferry. His stay was enjoyable by all accounts.

## CHAPTER 3

## MY CHRISTMAS DRESS

To Move or not to Move

My business had been thriving in Ireland, and in 2008, I launched my own brand of Caribbean food products called Taste of the Caribbean. I also started looking for a home in a more expensive neighbourhood with the desire to upgrade. Sean accompanied me on many house hunting expeditions to South Dublin which, according to Dubliners, was very exclusive. Eventually the reality of unreasonable mortgage loans and my precarious income hit, and I started looking farther away for a home. Sean spotted a mansion on the hill in his town of Tramore, Waterford County which was just a fraction of the price I would pay in Dublin for a similar property. One visit to view the home with the real estate agent was enough to set me on a campaign to win this house and sell my Dublin home. The home, originally built in the 1880s was a renovated historical site with an unobstructed view of Tramore Bay from the bedroom windows and attic. With three functioning fireplaces – one in the living room and two in the upstairs bedrooms, it was a rare dream.

I listed my home for sale, did a massive clean out and called a moving company. I was still negotiating the purchase of the house on the hill in Waterford County.

The real estate agent in Dublin made me panic… 'Prices have levelled out... Soon they'll start falling. Sell fast or else! There's a recession coming! Don't list the price too high, or else…'

After several weeks of walking on eggshells, my Dublin home had finally sold and I was forced to move out.

Unfortunately the new home purchase was not easy, so

Tiffany and I moved to a temporary residence until the dream home mortgage was finalized. That again was a nerve-wracking time since I felt homeless as a renter with my household belongings in storage. I decided to bid higher than the asking price just to speed things up. It was not a good decision in hind sight. The real estate market crashed a few months later and I was stuck with a large mortgage to pay as the market bottomed out.

Eventually the home was mine and we moved in with the massive task of unpacking while running a business and getting Tiffany settled in a new school, all at the same time.

'Mammy I bought a new house by the seaside,' I said, calling my mother, my biggest supporter over the years, to celebrate.

'A new house? Dat nice girl,' she said with gusto.

'You'll have to come and visit me sometime,' I continued.

'Of course,' she said. I wasn't sure if she fully understood where I lived and how she would get there.

During the year, moving and trying to run the business occupied my every waking hour. Tiffany was enrolled in a small village school in Fenor and was having adjustment problems. I stopped importing goods and looked for local facilities to manufacture my own sauces and spice blends. My product branding was changed and I signed up for new events and markets in the South East of Ireland. After a whirlwind year, a trip away to rest and recuperate was well deserved. Sean expressed disappointment at being left alone that Christmas. In fact he wasn't alone and would probably be negotiating back and forth for his children with his former wife. It was a good idea for me not to be part of that narrative. Sean became distant that year since I moved to Tramore and we didn't bond as we did before. He seemed to have a recent aversion to meeting and I had to make the difficult decision to part with the aloof and unconcerned partner, while still living in his small town and running into his friends daily. With no family support of my own, it was a challenging situation. A visit to Trinidad was just what the doctor ordered. We left for Trinidad on December 23rd and returned after the New Year.

## Slipping Fast

My mother was turning 77 in 2009 and her friend Kim was a few years her junior. Mammy and Kim had taught at the same secondary school in Port-of-Spain, Trinidad and remained friends long after retirement. Kim, from what I remembered, was soft spoken with a definite twinkle in her eyes. She made jokes sometimes, but always out of earshot when I was growing up. Kim was still very active and physically fit. The years had not been as kind to my mother after retirement. Her body was succumbing to arthritis in the knees and hands, but the worst affliction was the degeneration of her mind as a result of Alzheimer's disease. Mammy was losing her confidence and memory, and recognised the fact that she could no longer travel alone. She had loved to travel frequently in her younger years, jetting to the United States, England, or countries around the Caribbean. The whole year had passed without a trip and I suggested she and Kim come to visit me for Christmas. That year had been mediocre financially as the worldwide recession continued, so it was best for me to stay put for the holidays.

I had worked a three-day weekend at the Cork Christmas market on Grand Parade. The usual customers came around, as well as locals passing for samples out of habit. That Christmas all vendors were certainly feeling the brunt of the recession. People didn't have the buying power as in previous years. It wasn't easy to bear the cold, and remain cheerful all day, chatting with customers and trying to convince them that Caribbean style sauces made unique stocking stuffers! It was a strange idea too, when uncharacteristic snow was looming on the Irish horizon.

I baked Caribbean Christmas cakes spiked with rum and these were a big hit. When tied with red ribbon, cakes of all sizes made wonderful gifts. The cakes were in the shape of small loaves, some with fruits and blackened with molasses and browning, and other rum cakes without fruit.

Cork customers called them buns. 'Oh look at the little buns. Is there enough rum in them to get me drunk?'

'You would have to eat about five or six. I put one shot of rum in each cake!' I explained.

This was a source of amusement for many customers.

Since that weekend was a bit slow, I decided to work only two days the following week when Mammy arrived, so I could then spend the rest of the time preparing for Christmas.

My plan was to fly to the London Gatwick airport to meet my mother and Kim and fly back with them to Dublin. This meant renting a car in Waterford, driving to Dublin airport, leaving the car in long term parking, getting on an early jet out to Gatwick and taking the Gatwick shuttle in between terminals. I met them just as they left baggage claim and took them on the shuttle back to the other Gatwick terminal, so we could get our flight back to Dublin. After checking in, I tried without success to get them to eat lunch. It was going to be a long journey flying to Dublin followed by at least two and a half hours' drive to Waterford.

'We had something to eat on the plane', they protested.

'Yes, but that was hours ago!'

Mammy was extremely disoriented and nervous. She spilled all her tea on the table in the restaurant, and was already talking about going back to her house in Trinidad. It was going to be a very, very long day for me. We finally boarded the flight to Dublin and by the time we arrived, my two elderly companions were at their wits end with fatigue. As we drove to Waterford, Mammy got more and more agitated. The small roads were long and winding through every town. I knew every bend in the road, but for the unsuspecting traveller, it was grass, forests, trees, and bush… endless bush.

'You are taking me into the forest to kill me!' Mammy protested. 'Where are we going? Put me out now so I can take a taxi home!'

There was no stopping her, and Kim sat quietly, not knowing what to do. Mercifully, we got home in good time and we were able to get Mammy settled in Tiffany's room.

'Where am I?' she asked. 'How did I get here?'

I had to explain about three or four times how they flew to London, via Barbados, then from London to Dublin, then drove from Dublin to Tramore.

'Tra – More – Ray', Mammy kept saying. It was truly funny.

I unloaded the luggage, took back the rental car and retrieved my two-seater van from the parking lot of the rental car company. It was a solid 12 hours of travel for me.


Christmas Meeting

I'd recently participated in the filming of an episode of the

Irish Dragons Den and the following morning my initial appointment was scheduled with the Dragons who had pledged support in my business. Since the journey to collect my mother and Kim was so arduous, I decided to give myself a break from driving and take the train to Dublin. Kim was left in charge at the house and I showed her how to navigate around the kitchen. I left early to catch the train to Dublin. Luckily, parking was free at the Waterford train station and a spot not too far from the main entrance was available. The journey was ideal for collecting my thoughts and getting paperwork together for the meeting ahead. Having to refocus on business ideas, objectives and the future of the company was not an easy task.

As the train flew through Co. Kildare, my mobile phone started ringing. It was a call from the house. Kim was extremely flustered and worried because my mother was trying to run away and had attempted to open the front door many times to 'take a taxi back' to her house. She kept threatening to push Kim over. I felt helpless on the train. There was no turning back. I asked Kim to put Mammy on the phone so I could speak with her and reassure her that everything was OK. After about five minutes of talking, she calmed down a little and I promised to return home as early as possible. I knew my visit to Dublin could take all day, so I just prayed that Mammy would remain calm until I returned.

When the train arrived at Heuston Station, I tried to find my way to the Four Seasons Hotel in Ballsbridge. Not being able to see a ready bus, I hailed a taxi. Even though I had been really watching my pennies, I felt I had to make a good first impression and arrive on time. I forgot that Irish time was not necessarily American time though, and things were usually flexible. It was the first meeting with the Dragons after the filming in November, and I was not sure what to expect but remained hopeful. When I arrived, one Dragon was there, sipping tea and saying hello to every second person who passed. This millionaire was a tall man with a bald head and long nose, and ears pricked up like an elf's. He looked as if he was born in a suit. This conversation was certainly going to be interesting, I thought.

'She's going to make me rich with these Caribbean sauces!' he said to people passing by.

They all smiled and feigned acknowledgement. They didn't know what he was talking about, but smiled nevertheless. He was rich and famous, with businesses all over the country, and could say what he liked to these people.

Fifteen minutes later, my other mentor showed up and we chatted about the weather, the traffic, Christmas holidays, the programme, and maybe for twenty seconds about my business proposal and Caribbean sauces. Their conclusion was that nothing could be done until after Christmas.

Was that it… ?

I'd left a confused and disoriented mother and her frightened friend at home. Still exhausted from the previous day's adventure at the airport, I'd travelled three hours for a 15 minute meeting. There was no expensive lunch, gifts or celebration. One investor left to attend to important business. The other asked if I wanted to speak further at his office, since he had business to attend to over there. I thought maybe that would give me more opportunity to speak with him about my goal of getting his food distribution business to take my product into stores. I went along for the ride in his Bentley sports car and the butlers at the hotel proudly brought the car around to the doorway. It was my first trip in a Bentley sports car, so if nothing else, this made my day. I told him my mother was visiting and she had progressive Alzheimer's disease. He revealed that his mother was also afflicted with this condition.

I was shocked to see his tiny office upstairs in one of his stores. The place was being refurbished, but I had really expected something grander for a millionaire who collected Bentleys. A gigantic, old style Bentley was parked at one end of the little car park. The most splendid part of the office was a large boardroom table on which a collection of exquisite pottery stood. This was a product from another potential investment from the programme. We spoke for a short time and I got a few names and contacts, then it was time to go back to the train station.

'I'll call you a taxi', he said.

I could pretend to be a millionaire, but I wasn't taking taxis around the city. Going through the contents of my wallet and holding my breath, I found about €25. It was enough to pay the taxi. I let the driver know I was not new in the city, so he would not charge me the tourist rate. Mercifully, we reached the train station before my scheduled departure and I wondered what surprise was waiting for me at home.

Three hours later, when I got home, everyone was calm thankfully, and I set about fixing dinner. Kim and Mammy protested that they weren't hungry; however, when I placed the food in front of them, they ate ravenously. It was sad to watch the mental deterioration of someone who had been so grand and forthright in her peak. She really had become a child again.

Leo

In November, I'd started dating a man from Kildare County named Leo. He was a retired army man, and was running his own security firm with some business partners. He said he had been separated for years, and seemed like an interesting person. He had lived abroad, and had even witnessed battles. He was six feet tall and fit as a fiddle, with thinning fair hair, large bulging blue eyes and a bushy, blond moustache. I tried to read his intentions but failed. He seemed genuine but I had a nagging feeling that something was wrong with him, and hesitated to let him know where I lived or even to get into his large black Mercedes Benz.

He stopped at nothing to impress, by taking me to Waterford's finest restaurants. He really liked his food and had dabbled in cooking lessons. He even offered to help me set up at markets and food shows and soon started following me to events. I didn't know whether to be flattered or annoyed, but let him help when he wanted to. The truth was that I was happy to have a strong helper when I was packing up after a 10 or 12 hour work day.

Leo and I had planned an evening out two days before Christmas after my visitors were settled. He said I should bring a swimsuit and it was a surprise. I loved surprises and wondered what was in store. Leo had booked a massage for me at Solas Croi, the newly refurbished spa at the Brandon House Hotel in Wexford. We enjoyed the Jacuzzi and steam rooms followed by a massage and Thai dinner in Waterford City. It might have been romantic, except that I was not in love with him.

By 11:00 pm, I was totally fatigued and wanted to go straight home.

'I have guests at home,' I explained. 'I will have to go back soon to check on things. You know, make sure everything is fine.'

'Do you really have to go home?' he asked.

'Yes, I've neglected them long enough,' I said.

Leo delivered me to my front door. I could feel the tension

and annoyance oozing from his whole body. After putting in all this time and money, all I wanted to do was go home. It was enjoyable, but I didn't feel the same love and attraction I had felt for Sean. When we arrived at my door, I gave Leo a Christmas card which I had stored in my bag that afternoon. To which he responded by writing up a little card in front of me and handing it over. He seemed annoyed and so was I... a tit for tat.

Christmas in Tramore

I started cooking the Christmas meal a full day in advance, to prepare a wonderful feast for our visitors. Since my mother and Kim had to spend their vacation in a cold, old stone house, where the damp came in no matter how much the house was heated, the least I could do was make them a hearty meal.

I prepared roast turkey, ham leg, pork chops, roast lamb, macaroni and cheese pie, rice dishes and various salads. I made traditional black Christmas cake with rum and fruits, ice cream, fruit salad, and any other dish I could throw in for good measure. It was a meal for an extended family of 15, when in fact there were only four of us. Needless to say, we had food for days after Christmas.

Kim had been clamouring to go to the Catholic Church for Christmas mass. I could not deny them Christmas mass but only had a two-seater van. I decided to ask Sean the night before if he wouldn't mind taking us to his Church. I knew his routine well with his kids. After not speaking to him for weeks, it was a bit of a bold request, but one has to be bold sometimes. I did the polite thing and invited him to my home for Christmas dinner, offering an alternative to Christmas at his ex-wife's, if he wished.

On Christmas Day, we rose early and had a light breakfast. About ten minutes before Sean arrived to take us to church, I went to check on my mother who was dressing feverishly in her room. She was dressed in a beautiful, sleeveless blue and white dress with a light cotton shawl and silver sandals, with a silver handbag to match. The only problem was that it was 1ºC outside and the wind was howling, making it feel like -5ºC. In her mind, she was probably in the Caribbean on Christmas Day.

'Mammy, please, let's change everything and put on some warm clothes,' I begged.

'But then people at church won't see my dress,' she said. Despite losing some of her memory, she hadn't lost the desire to dress up and look beautiful. It was ingrained in her from childhood. Her whole family loved to dress to impress, including my grandmother.

'They really don't need to see your dress Mammy. It's too cold outside,' I said.

It took some convincing for her to wear extra garments, like a sweater, trousers, socks and boots, and a winter coat. In the meantime, Sean had arrived and was waiting downstairs. He was clearly annoyed to drive me and my clan around on Christmas morning and I didn't want to delay him an extra minute. We piled in and drove to the Protestant church in Tramore, the one with the shorter steeple. Nobody was in sight for miles. The roadway was empty even though the sign said Mass at 10am, so we drove on to the Catholic Church, which was starting its second mass of the morning. Everyone made it a point to attend Christmas Mass in Tramore. The church goers slumped into a trance as the priest gave his sermon and I spent my time studying all the faces to see who looked familiar and who was new. With so much to take in, the sermon and the whole ceremony went along swiftly. I tried to listen to the priest on a few occasions, but he seemed to be talking to himself and the message was unclear. It was no small wonder that so many looked lost.

Suddenly there was a flurry of activity as the priest announced Holy Communion, signalling the conclusion of the mass. People stirred, got ready to receive the sacrament, and then left. Sean collected us and we were swiftly deposited at my front gate. He shrugged off my Christmas hug and said goodbye.

The Christmas menu was a hit with Kim and Mammy.

However, Tiffany noted my exhaustion and blurted out to them, 'You're having a Christmas holiday, but not my Mammy!'

After spending two days indoors, we needed a day out so I could keep my sanity. We rented a car and I took the girls to see the most recent 3-D movie. My mother and Kim shouted at the screen wearing their 3-D glasses, much to Tiffany's amusement. They really enjoyed the action film. The following day I decided to take them to Cork City for a quick visit. With the short daylight hours, I wanted to leave early in the morning, but we ended up setting out closer to midday.

'I want to shop at Marks and Spencer,' Mammy proclaimed. 'I want to buy dresses. I have lots of money.'

I knew she had money and had been burning to spend it on something for days. However, I had no energy for a shopping trip, and she couldn't walk very fast or for long distances.

As we drove to Cork, I pointed to various interesting places along the way. I had done that drive so many times while working at events I could do it with my eyes closed.

My mother kept blurting out driving instructions along the

way,

'Go so! I said go so!'

This was amusing since she'd never been to Cork before.

At Swan Lake near Midleton, the fog made the lake barely visible. As I pointed out the area, I noticed that Mammy was wearing her 3-D glasses from the movie the night before. She couldn't possibly have seen anything clearly. Kim was not wearing her glasses at all that day and must have left them at home, so she wasn't seeing clearly either. My sightseeing tour was a futile effort.

The following day, we went on an outing to Dublin. December 29th was Mammy's birthday and I wanted to show her the bright lights of Dublin City. It was a cold, dark day, making the drive very dull. When we finally parked at St Stephen's Green shopping centre, we had a light lunch. I had planned to walk around Grafton Street, an upscale pedestrian shopping street in Dublin, and show them a few sights in the city. However, that plan was short-lived since my mother complained about the cold within half a block, and refused to walk any further. I calmly retrieved the rental car and we went off to visit a friend in Finglas. There we had a home cooked dinner, then drove back to Tramore. It was not a happy birthday. My nerves were strained to the limit.

New Year's Eve

Leo resurfaced after Christmas and we planned to go out for New Year's Eve. I had dreamt of going on a date to a dinner dance on New Year's Eve, ringing in the year with bells, whistles and screams of 'Happy New Year'. This was going to be my one night off, for a change of scenery and fun. Leo made reservations at Clontarf Castle in Dublin, where we would go to the New Year's Eve party, then stay overnight. I zipped into Waterford City to look for a lovely dress for the evening and snapped up a beautiful silver mini from an independent boutique. Disliking shopping very much, I was happy to find something quickly. At Debenhams I bought a pair of beaded stilettos and a cylindrical silver handbag that matched the dress, and then swiftly returned home.

While packing my bags to leave for the night, Kim and Mammy showered me with advice on what I should wear.

'You must wear stockings. You can't have your legs out!' said Kim.

'That dress is too short. You should have chosen something else,' said Mammy.

'You can't wear g-string underwear,' said Mammy. 'That's so common and low class for a lady. I'll lend you one of my knickers.'

'Mammy, yours may be a bit too big for me.' I said. 'I'll use what I have.'

Tiffany couldn't stop laughing. It amused her to see the two Grannies react in chorus during my preparation for the outing.

I left Kim in charge of the home, with extra food in the refrigerator and ideas for what meals they could prepare the next day. Kim wanted to go for a walk around the small town and I agreed since she was very fit and needed some exercise. Free at last, Leo and I drove happily out of town. We were very excited about the upcoming night of fun. It was to be a large dinner/dance with hats and whistles, and an opportunity to stay overnight at Clontarf Castle. With the M9 motorway newly opened, the journey to Dublin was shorter than previous years. Reports of a pending heavy snowfall filled the airwaves, but not much had fallen by that time. We hoped to be safely tucked away at night in Clontarf Castle with nothing to worry about when the storm hit. We were on the M9, just passing the Kilcullen exit in County Kildare, when I got a call from my neighbour in Tramore.

Kim had fallen in front of the house. She couldn't walk, and they had called for the ambulance!

A Snowy Beginning

As soon as my neighbour broke the news about Kim's accident, I rang the house. Mammy said Kim went off walking on her own and should have stayed at home like the rest of them. Tiffany took the telephone and gave me details of the incident. The paramedics took Kim out of the house on a stretcher and my mother wondered where the emergency responders were taking her friend.

Since we were almost in Dublin, Leo and I decided to continue, with the intention of returning early next morning. I felt so guilty having a poor old woman, a visitor, come to my home and meet such disaster. I also felt guilty because I was not on site to take care of her. Was I being a bad mother? I felt three times guilty for leaving three 'children' unattended and wondered how I could ever enjoy my night away.

I called a local friend who agreed to accompany Kim to the emergency ward at Waterford Regional Hospital. Tiffany said she was making pasta for Granny and everything was under control.

By the time we checked in, we were exhausted after the news and long drive and took a nap, waking up just in time for the dinner and dance. Dressing up in our finest, we went to the ballroom to join the other guests. After years of neglect, Clontarf Castle had been renovated into a splendid four-star hotel. We enjoyed looking at the old suits of armour in the hallway and relics of the ancient castle which stood in the middle of the lobby.

We sat at a large round table with five other couples. By chance, two other mixed-race couples were seated at our table. This was a unique coincidence. The room was decorated with balloons and each couple received party favours, including a crown and a hat that said 'Happy New Year 2010'. We spoke with everyone and when the dance music started, took to the dance floor. Leo was not much of a dancer, but he tried to match my enthusiasm as I bounced around.

At midnight, everyone hugged and greeted each other, shouting 'Happy New Year!' It was a wonderful atmosphere, even though I kept thinking about the absent ones – Tiffany looking after Granny, and Kim alone at the hospital in a strange country. I would have to go back as soon as I could next morning. Outside it was snowing heavily, even more than ever before. The city was not equipped to clear snow from the streets and we were lucky to be indoors that night.  At 1am, I asked Leo if he wanted to dance one last dance and he looked relieved and exhausted.

We ate at the buffet breakfast in the beautiful, sky-lit atrium at 7 am. Surprisingly, the restaurant was crowded at that time. It seemed like some had never gone to bed. Not having much of an appetite, I picked at the meal and was anxious to leave; the warnings on the news were clear.

Taking highway N11 along the coast instead of attempting Carlow and Kildare County, we hoped road conditions would be better. However, the main roads were particularly bad in the Dun Laoghaire-Rathdown County area, with snow piled several centimetres deep as we drove through. The car's wheels were spinning in some places. The roads had not been cleared and only one lane was functional most of the way. We had to drive at snail's pace not to fly off the road. Only a few other brave fools were out, but I was determined to get back to Waterford to oversee the situation.

We didn't stop, but it still took three and a half hours on the motorway to reach Waterford, with some near misses and skids along the way. As we neared the city, I called the hospital to find out what was happening with Kim. A friendly voice informed me that she had just gotten out of surgery and her hip was replaced. I was not allowed to see her until visiting hours later that afternoon. The whole world had certainly turned topsy-turvy on my one night out.

Leo left me in Tramore and drove straight back to Dublin. I got home to find a mountain of dirty dishes and Tiffany and Granny gossiping quite happily. After clearing up the mess and cooking a meal, I made my way to the hospital. I was always anxious at hospitals, but felt that Kim who must have been especially nervous in this provincial hospital in a foreign country. She was resting comfortably and had been given pain killers. Three other patients shared the room with her, and two were quite talkative and entertaining. I hoped that gossiping with roommates would lift her spirits.

I tried to visit each day to follow her progress to recovery. In the meantime, her daughter in Trinidad was advised to come to Ireland for the journey back home with her. Kim was not supposed to travel for another three weeks and had to spend some time with a physiotherapist. This regional hospital was famous for hip replacement surgery. It was said that if one stayed around too long in the waiting room, he would be carted off to have a hip replaced. It was funny how this hospital accepted patients without knowing about their insurance coverage. They only asked about insurance several days after completing major surgery. Luckily my mother, in one of her good and sane moments, had thought to purchase travel insurance before the journey. And it was a Godsend under the circumstances.

The hospital was ready to discharge Kim, but I couldn't take care of her. We had a long flight of steps just to enter the front door. Kim couldn't walk and all of the bedrooms were on the second floor of the house. I was trying to get the business started again after the long Christmas break and asked if she could stay at the hospital to recover. They complained many times about a healthy person taking up a bed when they had emergency situations. Luckily she was allowed to stay until she was well enough to travel.

Since Kim couldn't use her ticket to return to Trinidad, I made arrangements to book her on a later flight. In the meantime, my mother had to go back to Trinidad too. Winter was no good for her and I wanted to start working again to pay bills. The dilemma was how she should travel alone to Trinidad. My brother and I decided to do a relay of sorts. I would ensure she boarded the plane to Barbados at Gatwick airport. Then he would fly to Barbados to meet her when she landed, in time to change airlines for Trinidad. Every flight had to be well timed. As I handed her over in a wheelchair in London, I kept asking the attendant to make sure she got on the airplane and didn't walk around the airport. She pretended to hit me, making all the attendants giggle. She declared she wasn't a child and didn't need assistance. As I flew back to Ireland, I had visions of my mother walking around Gatwick airport and not boarding that airline. I couldn't sleep until I knew she was safe and my brother had met her in the airport. I tried calling him numerous times, but of course he couldn't answer his mobile phone when he was flying.

Finally, the next day, I got news that all was well and

Mammy was back at her home. But her trip wasn't without drama. Mammy was found wandering outside the airport in Barbados because she thought she had arrived home. What an ordeal we'd all experienced, and it was such a relief to know she was safely in her house and familiar surroundings.

Now it was time to see Kim safely back to Trinidad. Her daughter, Kezianne was to fly to Dublin and I gave her directions for getting the J. J. Kavanagh airport shuttle all the way to Tramore. On the morning she arrived, I was at the bank and supermarket and poor Kezianne arrived in Tramore at 12:00 pm instead of the later 1:00 pm arrival time that I anticipated. Her mobile phone received no signal in Ireland and a young store clerk at a convenience store allowed Kezianne to call on her cell phone. I rushed back to find Kezianne in tears. It was really heartbreaking because I knew she'd endured a long journey. But we got settled, enjoyed something to eat, and then went to visit Kim at the hospital. It was a good reunion.

I asked Leo if he would take Kim and Kezianne from the Waterford hospital to Dublin Airport for me since he owned a big car and Kim's leg needed to stay extended. At first he agreed to be the chauffeur, but then he mysteriously stopped calling and disappeared. I decided to rent a car and do the driving myself. When we reached the airport, we were able to get a wheelchair at the entrance to the airport departure lounge. I left my passengers to check in and swiftly drove back to Waterford. Kim and Kezianne were flying to London to rest for a few days with relatives before taking the long flight back to Trinidad. It was a bittersweet departure from Ireland, after a vacation gone all wrong…

## Chapter 4

## POKE IN DE CALLALOO

Granny's Mean

My mother continued to live alone at her house in Diego Martin. It was her familiar environment. My father lived with his partner in Barataria. With elderly parents, I always felt a bit guilty living thousands of miles away and not being able to help them. I decided to travel to Trinidad on holidays for Carnival 2010 to follow up on my mother who experienced some trauma on the long journeys to and from Ireland at Christmas time. I pulled Tiffany out of school, as usual, with the firm belief that travel was education. Mammy settled ever so slightly when she returned to her home environment, but my father was suffering from cancer. I stayed with Mammy in Diego Martin and made regular visits to see Pops.

My mother had become more argumentative and suspicious as time went on. One day, I overheard Khadir with my other nephews in the garage complaining about their grandmother.

'Granny pinched me!'

'Yeah, and she hit me ...'

'Uh huh, and she made a monkey face at me!'

'Granny's mean!'

'I don't like Granny!'

They seemed to be plotting a mutiny against poor old Granny.

Alzheimer's disease caused my mother to be violent and

argumentative. She insulted everyone in her path. Looking at Tiffany, she told me, 'Why don't you comb dat chil' hair? Do somethin' with yuh own hair. It's a mess. Yuh face looks so greasy, put a little powder on it nah.'

Mammy slowly but surely estranged some of her best friends with her neurotic behaviour, accusing them of stealing her belongings and other transgressions. Her verbal and small physical attacks on family and friends also increased. Her friend Leonore who used to visit to play scrabble was chased off with insults and accusations. One of her long time friends, Petra from Couva was also accused of stealing her clothing and kitchenware. Mammy even called me while I lived in Ireland, to complain about Petra stealing her clothes, and I believed her.

My mother began hiding everything from the thieves and the friends who stole. She would wrap jewellery in tissue paper and hide it in between linen in drawers and closets. New underwear was hidden in odd places. The styrotex foam trays from packets of chicken and old margarine containers were washed and saved. Even full boxes of juices were hidden behind books on the book shelf until they began to burst open attracting flies and cockroaches, increasing the pest problem at the house. Half eaten rotis, hundred dollar bills, bags of rice … everything was worth hiding from 'THE PEOPLE'.

On most of my visits home for vacation, the first few days were spent cleaning and finding the stashes of hidden goods and money around the home. A cardboard barrel once used to ship goods from New York City was used for storage and hiding. The barrel took a coveted spot in corner of the dining room covered over gingerly with a beautiful table cloth. It was a gold mine for finding hidden dried food stuff, coveted pots and pans, or a prized knife wrapped in tissue. Mammy hid everything. Under the mattress in her bedroom, I found decades old calendars and newspapers, as well as odds and ends of clothing, all fit for disposal.

When I cleaned, it was necessary to hide all the items being removed from the house for disposal. She once threatened to beat me up because I carried garbage bags with old bath mats and towels to the curb for the rubbish truck to take them away. With at threat to 'chop me up', she dragged the garbage bags back into the house and proceeded to unpack everything.

'How dare you come from away and try to throw away my things! Go back where you came from!' she shouted, filled with rage and a cutlass in her hand.

I was genuinely afraid, because her rage was so strong. I admitted defeat that day and looked for another strategy.

One day, Brent and I coordinated to have one of us remove Mammy from the house with the promise of going to Macqueripe for a 'sea bath', while the other carted away bags of waste that were out of site at the back of the house. On that occasion the strategy worked and we knew she would never miss the items that were removed. It was unbelievable how much plotting and scheming was necessary to clean the home in which our mother lived, so she wouldn't cause harm to herself.


Carnival Time

My father had been suffering from cancer at that time and the cancer seemed to spread from the prostate gland to the colon. He underwent radiation and chemotherapy which made him extremely ill and weak. We received reports of him fainting on the tennis court while meeting with friends. My father appeared withered and just a shadow of the tall, strong man I used to know as a young child and adult. After seeing him, Colette and I both felt he was on his last days and might not have been able to hold on much longer. During Carnival celebrations he used to stand for hours looking at the parade and socializing with friends in the hot sun. It was not the same that year. He could hardly walk to Adam Smith Square where they set up a picnic with food and drinks under the shady trees. He sat in the shade most of the day without seeing the all-day Carnival parade for fear of experiencing a fainting spell. When our band passed on Ariapita Avenue near Adam Smith Square, Colette and I left the group in our costumes to visit with Daddy, show him our costumes and have lunch. We knew he would have prepared food and drinks for us, as in previous years and would expect us to visit.

What a pitiful sight he was. We tried to take photographs and keep conversation light and happy to prevent ourselves from crying. It was bad enough grappling with Mammy and her violent tendencies. But then to see my Pops so weak and trying his best to remain jovial broke my heart. We returned to Ireland wondering if we would ever see him again.

Getting the News

Pops received chemotherapy again and suffered from a host of side effects. One day in spring while merchandising my Caribbean products at a big supermarket in Lucan, near Dublin, my brother called from the hospital in Port-of-Spain to say our dad was not doing very well. Pops came on the phone but could barely speak.

'Pops, you're giving us a scare. You have to stay well OK,' I said. 'I'm really starting to worry about you.'

He couldn't say much. He just muttered in agreement and gave the phone back to Brent. I knew something was drastically wrong. He would usually attempt a short conversation and give a little joke when he could. After hearing his faltering speech, I realised he must have been in severe pain. I couldn't maintain my composure and packed immediately to leave for the day. It wasn't possible to speak to consumers about the joys of Caribbean sauces when all I wanted to do was cry.

I tried calling Pop's cell phone the next day but there was no answer. Two days later, I got the ill-fated news that Pops passed away at the hospital. We all expected this news one day. He was in pain for over a year, with continuous fainting spells making driving and daily life unbearable. His death, however, was still a shock for all of us. I wailed and cried for an hour then decided to reach out to my sister, Colette who was living in Atlanta, Georgia at the time. We spoke back and forth during the week leading up to this moment and she said she knew it was the end when he was admitted to hospital.

I kept thinking there was hope against hope in his fight against cancer. He always spoke fondly of one of his cousins from Tobago who received chemotherapy and was able to bounce back to life. In the end, his body was weak and finally collapsed. After crying again and feeling sorry for myself, I was forced to snap out of the self-imposed misery and look for plane tickets to Trinidad for the funeral.

Brent was the only sibling based in Trinidad with the brunt of the responsibility of identifying the body at the hospital and contacting the funeral home to make all arrangements. He told us the grisly story how the hospital never called to let him know our father had died the previous day. He only found out when he arrived during visiting hours the next day and saw that the bed was empty. When he enquired at the staff desk, they told him to go to the morgue to identify the body. I could only imagine his pain at that point in time. The horror and indignity of the whole process was beyond comprehension.

Brent waited for Colette and me to book our flights to Trinidad in order to determine the best date for the funeral. He also wanted to get some input on the order of the funeral service. Colette wanted to present a eulogy and set about writing one immediately. I was going to sing a religious song of significance and hoped my voice wouldn't crack mid-song from grief.

Colette was a little upset that she wasn't in Trinidad to participate in minute details of the funeral planning. However, by the time we arrived in Trinidad, everything for the funeral would already be in place. Brent contacted the funeral home, selected a casket, and made reservations at the St. James crematorium. The funeral home assisted in making public announcements and designing the program. Pops wisely put aside an insurance policy to cover funeral expenses, so everything was arranged. Our cousins from the United States also made arrangements to fly to Trinidad for their Uncle Kenneth's funeral. He was their favourite uncle who had stood by his sister and her brood through thick and thin when they were young.

Three days after getting the news that Daddy had died, Tiffany and I left Tramore, heading first to Dublin, then flying to London, Gatwick. I felt weak from crying and could barely contain my grief. The immigration officer in Gatwick was new and in training with a supervisor breathing down his neck. He interrogated me continuously about why I was coming to the UK and how long I would be staying, which I found irritating. I didn't have the patience to answer what I considered useless interrogation. I was only passing through their airport. Why couldn't he read my mind and feel my pain? We spent a few hours in the airport before getting on a flight to Port-of-Spain, Trinidad. Mercifully, the time passed swiftly and before I knew it, all siblings were assembled the next day at my mother's house in Diamond Vale, Diego

Martin.

We went to the funeral home for the final arrangements and to discuss the ceremony which was scheduled for the following day. The attendant said he would bring out Pops' body for us to see. I questioned how I was going to handle seeing him. It was one thing to hear about a dead parent, but another to actually see him. Slowly, slowly the attendant rolled the casket towards us for inspection. The staff may have been quite proud of their work in preparing the dead for funerals, and I knew I would have to push myself to show appreciation for a job well done. But, did I dare look? I gulped with fear. How could Pops be in this box? How was it possible? As the tears rolled down my face, the attendant opened the casket and it took all the courage I could find to look.

There lay Pops, motionless. He was dressed in a formal suit with a tie. His skin looked ashy and somewhat powdery with makeup. I felt numb from head to toe. I still couldn't believe it was actually true. I didn't want to believe he was dead. But, as the saying goes, 'Seeing is believing' and I needed to believe. I could not touch him. All I could do was look. He used to be a big stocky man, but with the ravages of cancer, Pops looked like a mere skeleton. Cancer was certainly the worst possible affliction on earth. Despite the various treatments of chemotherapy and radiation, nothing halted its effects. I was hoping with all my heart for a miracle to heal him, but this was not to be.

'Thanks so much for taking care of him,' I said to the undertaker sobbing quietly. 'He looks fine in his suit.'

Brent and Colette nodded quietly in agreement. It was all we could say. The attendant then wheeled his body back to the storage facilities. We looked at the final order of service for the program before they sent it to print. We needed to be strong for each other that day. Colette moaned again because all the arrangements were made without her input.

'Well, we don't live in Trinidad,' I said. 'What did you expect? Why should Brent wait for us to arrive before planning the funeral? I don't think it would have made much of a difference. He was right to go ahead.'

'Well I wanted to have an input,' she complained. I started crying again as the funeral home manager reviewed the program with us.

Brent, the youngest in our family, was a man of few words. He was at least six feet tall, with an ample belly and a calm demeanour. He remained calm no matter what was happening. He gave the final cheque to the funeral home, and we left. The funeral was scheduled the following morning at St Michael's and All Angels Anglican Church on Wendy Fitzwilliams Boulevard in Diamond Vale. It was the church we attended as children. We then planned to go to the St. James Crematorium for a short ceremony before Daddy would be cremated. After, we would entertain close friends and family with some finger food and drinks at Pops' home in Barataria. It was the part of the funeral many looked forward to: socializing, eating and drinking. Funerals and weddings were social events. Pops complained months before his death that he attended too many friends' funerals and wished for happier opportunities to socialize.

Funeral Service for Poke

The next day we arrived early at the church before the funeral home was scheduled to bring the casket. Tiffany, Colette, my mother and I dressed early and came to the church to take in the scene. The church was decorated for the weekend services so plants and flowers were everywhere. I told Mammy that Pops had died, but she showed no emotion. We weren't quite sure if she understood what was going on and why we were black dresses that morning. She enjoyed dressing up and going out, so perhaps it was just another outing for her. When the funeral home brought the casket, they placed it near the main entrance and asked if we wanted the top to be opened. I didn't object. It was one way for visitors to pay their last respects.

The church looked the same as when we were growing up. The polished grey concrete floors, cherry-brown wooden pews, and concrete grey-brick side walls open to the top to let in fresh air remained the same. Modern architecture abounded with concrete and steel posts. Gaps in the walls were created with metal gratings to let in more air. The altar formed an island near the back of the church. The priest was a young fellow I'd never seen before. However, I left Trinidad at least 18 years before, and shouldn't have expected anything to stay the same as when I left. I wondered about Father Gray, the priest we knew when we were growing up. Why couldn't he officiate at Pops' funeral? I heard he was still alive and serving in other parishes at the time.

Daddy was a retired secondary school teacher and Principal and he was actively involved in the Lions Club, providing community service for years. He was also an avid tennis player since his university days. This meant that the church was crowded with people from all walks of life. The members of his Lions Chapter wanted to officiate as pall bearers and also give a speech at the service. We omitted adding them to the program, so this was a matter of contention. Many past pupils, teachers and staff of the various schools where Pops taught History and English, and officiated as Principal were in attendance. Some of their faces were familiar since many of our family friends over the decades were teachers. This usually happened in a household where both parents were educators. I also taught for a brief period at the school where Pops was Principal and so I walked around the church briefly, greeting some of the teachers from back in the good old days. I extended my gratitude for their coming to pay respects on that sombre day. However, I didn't quite know what more to say.

'Thanks for coming. Good to see you.'

Daddy got the nickname of 'Pork in the Callaloo' shortened to 'Poke' from an early age. People spoke about 'Poke' affectionately as they assembled for the funeral. Some of his tennis buddies from Public Servants Association tennis courts and the Diamond Vale courts also attended the service. During a very sick period following chemotherapy, Pops still found the energy to go on the tennis court, because he was passionate about the sport. He arranged his 75th birthday party at a tennis court, inviting some of his tennis friends to eat and drink after 'hitting some balls', as the slang went. There was no stopping him, until one time we got a phone call to say he collapsed on the court and an ambulance was called to take him to the hospital. I could do nothing living thousands of miles away. Taking away his socializing at the tennis court was like killing him swiftly.

As family and friends poured in the church, they brought flowers and laid them near the casket. My cousin Marianna who flew in from New York City the day before, stood near the entrance. Marianna may have been Pops' favourite niece. He used to spend many a summer in New York hanging out with friends at her house. She cried when she saw his whittled body in the casket and patted his chest for comfort. She stood a long time at his side crying and praying. Seeing her reaction made me heart broken and I cried even more. Another cousin, Sandra, also came from New York and her brother, Linford, the only boy in their family flew in from Maryland. He was over six feet tall and built like a basket-ball athlete. He had a happy-go-lucky character and enjoyed teasing. Charlene, the youngest girl in their family and close in age to Colette and me arrived from Maryland too. She resembled her mother who was my dad's sister. Katy, their only sibling residing in Trinidad did not speak to her siblings because of a family feud over inheritance. It was a fight we did not understand.

I hugged a few people who came into the church and after a while became too overwhelmed. I decided to sit quietly up front with my mother and Tiffany, and prepare mentally for the service when I would sing my song. The heat and humidity bore down on us that morning. My mother who was 77 at the time looked around the church saying hello to a few people who approached to show their respects.

Our parents were separated since I left high school and Mammy had rarely spoken to Pops over the years. His passing away may not have been significant to her, and I wasn't sure if she understood what was going on that morning and who had died. People were coming to her with words of comfort and all she would do was smile at them without quite recognising them. It was hard to believe people still didn't recognise her signs and symptoms of Alzheimer's disease. As the funeral began the room temperature seemed to rise steadily with the approaching noon hour. The young priest gave a very inspiring, thought-provoking sermon without really knowing our father. His lecture was calming. When my turn came to sing, however, all the nervousness returned. I sang a cappella and tried not to choke on my tears. I wanted to sing in full voice to make Pops proud.

I sang two verses of Amazing Grace, and the song passed mercifully quickly and then I was able sit down and relax. Tiffany read from the New Testament Bible and Colette did a stellar job reading her eulogy.

She described Pops' childhood and also how he taught her in high school. She got no special favours as a student in his class, and was sometimes passed over when he selected students to answer questions. Pops' community involvement, passion for tennis, love of family, and love of food were discussed during the eulogy. He used to say he would only go to church for weddings and funerals. These outings had become a popular social activity for people like him in their 70's.

At the end of the service we processed through the church and well wishers showed their sympathy. We drove in procession in my mother's car to the crematorium, and sat in the front row of the chapel. There, Daddy's cousin Janice officiated, and her daughters who sang professionally, performed a number of Gospel pieces as a farewell to their Uncle. The celebrant said a few words and then announced the body would be taken to a special room for cremation and we would not be allowed in that room. He then asked who would keep the crucifix that decorated the top of the casket.

My mother who hadn't said a word during the whole funeral service, at that point put out her hand immediately and said,

'I will keep it!'

We were surprised at this sudden awakening, and of course let her have it. The crucifix would most likely get hidden somewhere in the house with all the other lost objects she was hiding from 'The PEOPLE'. He handed her the small plastic crucifix and staff wheeled the casket out of the chapel. It was then I broke down in tears again. The thought of Pops being burnt up in an incinerator was too much to fathom. I started bawling and crying and nobody could console me.

I dragged myself unwillingly to the corridor in time to see the men wheel the casket into the back room and shut the door. I hung onto Brent's arm and wept. Just then Daddy's partner, who was also in the crowd, started crying loudly. My mother looked around asking why we were crying and if Daddy was dead.

'Kenneth dead? Eh? He dead?'

At that point she realised he was dead and kept asking questions. It took a while for me to calm down and regain self-control. The closing of that door was like the final goodbye. His body would be burned beyond recognition. He was going to be reduced to dust. It was a very difficult fact to accept.

'Come on Lindy, let's leave,' said Colette. 'I'll take Mammy and Tiffany home and then we can go to Daddy's place in Barataria for the repass.'

That was a good idea. There was no point having them drive around all day. The morning outing was long enough. Many family members and old friends left the crematorium to head to Barataria for the repass.

The visit to Trinidad was bittersweet, a celebration of my father's life and a chance to reunite with cousins who had flown in from the United States for the funeral. We scattered my father's ashes at the ancestral home of the James' in St. Cecelia, Tobago. He would have liked that.

Alas, it was time to say farewell knowing very well my cousins, the Trini Expats, would all go our separate ways, perhaps never to see each other again for many years. We would be flying back to our respective homes: New York, Washington D.C., Maryland, Atlanta, and Dublin.

CHAPTER 5

HOME AGAIN

2011 Carnival

Recession in Ireland in 2009 and 2010 presented daunting challenges that made it difficult to continue running my business profitably. Consequently, I decided to move back to Canada to make a fresh start after an extended absence. It was the end of December 2010, the middle of winter and a tough time for settling in a new city. This was the time when Tiffany and I left Ireland for Toronto, Canada. To escape the frigid temperatures, we took a vacation to Trinidad for Carnival; a welcome relief from the cold weather and isolation in the new city.

In the years following her retirement my mother held the position of President of the Senior Achievers Association, a group consisting primarily of retirees who still had a zest for life. Mammy had been involved in planning various parties and outings. Even after she had left her post with the Association and showed signs of Alzheimer's, Colette and I took turns in taking her to the annual Senior Achievers Carnival party over the years. On my trip back to Trinidad, I planned to take her that Carnival Sunday afternoon to the dance, where she could have fun with her peers. Mammy's car was at the repair shop for many days and she couldn't drive. Brent promised to give us a ride to the party and had made arrangements for a friend to bring us home. Unable to see her car in the garage, my mother became very upset and decided to walk to the mechanic's shop that Sunday morning.

Despite my best efforts there was nothing that I could say or do to prevent her from making the trek in the blazing sun. I took her hand to guide her back into the house but she was very strong and very angry. She threatened to punch me and

I had to let her go. With a stick in one hand and a mission firmly cemented in her head she made her way down the road to the mechanic's shop where her car was being repaired. That morning she walked with energy, commitment and determination that she hadn't displayed in a very long time.

The mechanic conducted his business from his front yard. On that very day, the residents on the street were hosting a big Carnival Breakfast street party to mark the occasion. My concern was that the mechanic had some vicious guard dogs in his yard. Given the potential for a disaster to unfold, I prayed that he had fenced them in at the back of the property since many people would be on the street that morning. If my mother attempted to enter his yard, those animals would surely tear her to bits. Mammy was wearing a black sleeveless blouse with patterns and a pair of white leggings. This outfit was fine for the house but not suitable for walking down the street. However, she was determined to go just the way she was and there was nothing I could do to stop her.

'That mechanic better have my car ready,' she threatened. 'He's had it for days now!'

I tried calling my brother on his cell phone to look out for Mammy since he was at the street party. She used to say Brent was 'Her son in whom she was well pleased'. Colette and I were the wayward women who went astray and lived abroad. So, I called her 'son in whom she was well pleased' to find his mother and bring her safely home so she wouldn't get lost in the crowds at the street party.

After about half an hour I wasn't able to reach him. However, I saw Mammy walking back up the street full of energy like when she left. She said she hadn't seen the mechanic and there was too much noise. What a relief; she was back in one piece.

I served her some lunch and an ice cold drink. She would have been dehydrated after her walk in the hot sun, but she wouldn't really have noticed. Eventually Brent returned home to take us to the seniors' dance.

'OK Mammy, it's time to get changed for the party,' I said, hoping she would get out of the transparent leggings and wear something different.'

'Changed for what?' she asked puzzled.

'Remember you're going to the party this afternoon. It's your favourite Carnival Dance,' I told her. 'Time to change your clothes.'

'I'm not changing my clothes,' she said stubbornly.

'Yes you are,' I said. 'You can't go in the same clothes you wore this morning.'

I coaxed and pleaded for about fifteen minutes, but she refused to change. Eventually I gave up. It wasn't worth the fight. A great deal of patience is needed with someone suffering from Alzheimer's disease and I was not really blessed with the patience to say the same thing repeatedly.

'Where are we going?' she asked half an hour later.

'We're going to the Senior Achievers Carnival Dance,' I said, for the umpteenth time. 'That's your favourite Carnival party. You'll get to dance and see all your friends.'

We were forced to explain the same thing quite a few times in the car on the way to the event. When we arrived, Mammy walked in slowly through the gates as I gave our tickets.

'Hi Gloria, how are you?' asked a few elderly ladies and gentlemen.

'Fine thanks,' my mother answered, although I got the impression she didn't really know who these people were.

Even though we arrived a few minutes early, many of the over 70s patrons were already at the venue reserving their tables and chairs. Young people would arrive fashionably late to events, but the elderly were always early because they were worried about not having anywhere to sit down. Why sit when you're coming to a dance? Well, if you have arthritis in the knees, as was Mammy's case, a seat was vital. I was lucky to see two empty chairs at a table near the entrance as soon as we walked in. Mr. and Mrs. O'Dowd, our childhood friends occupied two seats at the table, so I was happy to see them and chat a little. They gave Mammy a frigid stare and cold shoulder, and I felt some tension. She said hello with a big smile, but I doubted she recognised them. Mammy must have slighted them in the past but I didn't know the story. Surely they recognised she was not mentally stable. They were of sound mind just like most of the party goers. Was my mother the only one suffering from a form of dementia at that event? If the elderly were not able to recognise dementia in their peers, well other members of the public would surely be no better. Perhaps people suffering from all forms of dementia were locked away and not allowed by their families to go out and have fun.

The Soca music was blaring and my mother got onto the dance floor immediately, joining three other dancing souls. Arthritis or not in her knocking knees, she didn't seem to mind. I saved her seat for her with a bag and spoke to a few of the friends around. She came to sit for a while and I brought some of the food and drinks which were being served so she could eat and be refreshed.

I had asked an old friend to collect us at 4:30 pm in the afternoon. This gave Mammy at least two and a half hours of dance time. There was no stopping her. She did her two-step dance to almost every calypso the DJ played, and only sat down briefly to have some refreshments. The DJ played old favourites from the 70s and 80s and years before, and this pleased the crowd immensely. Mammy sometimes danced with the other folks, and sometimes alone. Eventually I got a call from my friend saying she was close to the venue and we should stand outside. The dance hall was sweltering hot with many large fans, but the intense heat was wearing me out and I was seated half the time.

At last we returned home and Mammy got ready for bed. She was tired and needed no coaxing to have a shower and get dressed for bed.

'Ooh mih knees hurting mih,' she said in a bit of pain. 'Why mih foot hurtin' so much.'

'That's because you danced a lot at the party,' I explained. 'You enjoyed the Soca music so much, you hardly sat down!'

'Party? What party? I went to a party?' she asked.


Colette Moves Back

Colette was bored with her situation in Atlanta, and decided to move back home to Trinidad and Tobago. She packed lock, stock, and barrel in 2011 with her son Khadir and took up residence in Gloria's house. At first, it seemed like the best idea. She would be able to keep an eye on my mother to ensure she didn't harm herself as the Alzheimer's disease continued to affect mind and body.

This decision proved to be a nightmare. My mother was quite attached to her car and after a while she started fighting and challenging anyone who asked to use it. Colette had to get a job as soon as possible and get her own vehicle.

She managed to get a position overseeing a private elementary school for students with learning disabilities. Having a Masters degree in Early Childhood education and curriculum development, this role gave her an opportunity to use her skills. She had to rise early every morning and leave Khadir to dress himself and walk to the Diamond Vale Primary School just a few blocks away.

Colette cleaned the house and renovated many areas that were in varying stages of disrepair. The problem of termites in the foundation and roof had to be solved with intense treatment. The family's piano which was being devoured by termites, and some other furniture had to be removed. Mammy had accumulated clothing, kitchen ware, trinkets and many disposable items as she became obsessive and lived alone. One had to fight her to clear debris out of the house. Colette also brought all her furniture and household belongings to be housed somewhere. Her task was to sort through everything in the house and remove old or derelict items without our mother knowing.

On many occasions, my mother would say, 'Go back wherever you came from. Stop throwing away my things! I'll knock you over if you throw away my things!'

Redecorating the house was a gruelling task, but Colette managed to bring the home back to its former glory.

Many verbal fights ensued with my mother threatening my sister physically. Colette called to tell me she had hidden all the knives in the house in a place where my mother could never find them. This confused Mammy, when she looked high and low and couldn't find a knife. Colette would say she had to sleep with one eye open because Mammy walked around at night making mischief. Another point of contention was that Colette had a lock installed on her bedroom door. Colette occupied our childhood bedroom. Since she kept her valuables in this bedroom, she didn't want our mother rummaging through her belongings or misplacing important documents. Before she went to work, Colette was sure to lock the door. This irritated Mammy who complained that it was her house and she should be allowed to enter any room that she wanted.

One day, Mammy removed the louvres at the south side of this bedroom which backed into the former music room. She then climbed into Colette's room and unlocked the door so she could access the bedroom. This enraged Colette when she returned from work that day to see the door wide open and a few items moved out of place. My mother was in the garden tending to her plants and had completely forgotten that she climbed into the room, leaving the tell tale louvres on the floor beside the window. Another day, the neighbour told Colette that Mammy came over to ask her grandson, Giovanni to climb through the window to open the locked door. That weekend, Colette arranged with a handyman to completely seal that back window with concrete blocks while Mammy was out. She then reinstalled the curtain over the area. There was a lot of fretting and threatening when the agile Mammy found the area permanently sealed and she couldn't climb in.

I heard that my mother mistook Khadir for her big brother Wallace, as her mind played tricks on her. Khadir may have resembled Wallace in his childhood days. My mother attempted to fight with Khadir and hit him the way she used to fight with her big brother when he teased her. Unfortunately, Khadir couldn't understand why his Granny, would treat him so badly. One day she even threatened to chop him. Colette started waking Khadir early in the morning before she left for work to take him to the neighbour's house opposite, where he would wait in safety until it was time to walk to school.

After following this routine for a few weeks, and having to keep an eye on my mother on weekends, Colette felt it was too stressful for her young son. She made the tough decision to send him back to South Carolina in the United States, where he could be raised by his father and stepmother. This was not an easy choice, but since our mother's behaviour was unpredictable, it made no sense to risk her child's life. With a lot of tears and mourning, she packed all his things and shipped him out. He was going to miss his mother, but he was glad to get away from his grandmother who treated him badly. Colette was then left alone with Mammy and the troubles continued.

Colette was not able to continue working at the school and after the employment situation unravelled, she decided to move back to the Unites States. Our mother was then left temporarily in her home with some supervision from Brent on weekends and hired helpers came to the house to check in on her during the week.


No More Driving

My mother would spend time milling around her home which she knew well, but we didn't trust her driving around town. She was, however, very attached to her car. Several copies of the car keys and house keys were made so my brother and the neighbour could keep copies in case Mammy locked herself out. She was also equipped with a cell phone to call Brent if there was an emergency. Poor Brent was bombarded with calls while in meetings or on the road. He could get a call asking where she was supposed to be going to, and other strange questions. I even got a call in Ireland to ask where she was going. It was comical. We should have been worried about her driving, but for a time we were not bothered.

The feeling was that she wouldn't go far. Her favourite drive was to a roti shop on the Diego Martin Main Road (roti – wrapped sandwich with a curried meat or vegetable filling) and back through Diamond Vale to get home.

During a visit to Trinidad, she asked me if I wanted a roti and proceeded to drive to her favourite place. Her driving was slightly erratic at times and I had to block my eyes with my hands in fear, but we made it to the destination unscathed. My mother drove skilfully into the little parking space in front of the roti shop and walked through the wide open wooden doors like she owned the shop.

During one such visit, it was 11:30 am and a few patrons were on site buying their lunch. The attendants at the counter smiled when they saw Ms Gloria. She boasted to them that I was her daughter visiting from 'the cold' and they smiled gleefully as my mother ordered bone chicken rotis.

'They know me here,' she told me. I found out later that they knew her so well, that sometimes she came with short change like $5 to purchase a $15 roti, but they forgave her because she was an old regular and they possibly recognised she suffered from a form of dementia.

Backing the car out onto the Diego Martin Main Road after shopping was tricky for any driver, but Mammy drove with confidence and screamed at anyone who challenged her.

'Let him try to drive over me. Go over me!' she would yell at the blowing car horns.

Like a homing pigeon, and by a miracle in my opinion, she would get easily through a side road into Diamond Vale and back to her house.

My cousin, Richy warned us about my mother's driving saying she was a danger to herself and the general public. As we tried to wean Mammy away from her car and driving on the roads, Colette started giving her the wrong car keys. This trick enraged Mammy as she would try to open the car and the keys would not work. She would then complain to Colette that the keys were not working and Colette would say she couldn't understand why. This was the ultimate deceit, but we were afraid she would get into an accident while driving.

My mother had also become stingy with her car when we visited on vacation. She proclaimed loudly that nobody could use her car and we had to go back wherever we came from or get our own car. Since her vehicle was parked in the garage most of the time, I attempted to use it one day to go out for a swim, and she threatened to chop me. She snatched the keys which were usually placed in a green glass bowl on top of the fridge and ran with them to her bedroom. I followed in hot pursuit and watched her put the keys in a jewellery box on the dressing table. I then walked away quickly before she could realise I knew where the keys were hidden. Just as I predicted, within half an hour, she had forgotten where the keys were hidden. I took the keys from the jewellery box and kept them in my own room. When I asked Mammy where I could find the car keys, she headed for the glass bowl on top of the fridge which was the usual resting place for the keys. Not finding them, she raised the alarm and looked all around the house frantically.

'Where are my car keys? Where are my keys? I have to go out and buy a roti! Lindy where are my keys?' she asked.

'Well, I'm sure they are wherever you left them,' I would say in mischief. It takes two to Tango and she loved mischief.

When we felt she could no longer care for herself, I hid the car keys and never gave them back. It was a terrible thing to do and I felt guilty. It was so sad to watch as my mother bawled like a baby, not being able to find her car keys. Her independence was stripped away abruptly. She loved driving her car and would recognise that vehicle long into the final stages of Alzheimer's disease.

Home Care

My mother cooked simple meals for herself and Brent would buy groceries delivering them to the house every week. In hindsight, I wondered how we trusted her not to destroy the house with her cooking. Every time I called her to ask what she had cooked, she would say chicken and rice. I knew she'd wake up early to prepare her breakfast which was usually some form of sausage and meat, with toast and a cup of tea. One day, the neighbour opposite, Aunty Beris, called Brent to say that she smelled something burning and found Mammy in the yard watering plants while a pot of food burned to charcoal inside.

We hired a lady to come to the house a few days a week to clean the home and cook a meal for my mother. The housekeeper was responsible for making sure my mother didn't harm herself or destroy her house. Without regular supervision, however, the caregiver took advantage of the situation and this did not work. The house was reduced to a rat invested residence putting my mother's life in danger. We then hired a mother and daughter team who took turns in coming to the house Monday to Friday, again to clean and cook a meal, making sure my mother ate. They too took advantage of the old lady and her belongings, bringing at least three children to eat big meals at my mother's expense, and leaving my brother wondering why the groceries were being depleted so quickly every week.

One morning, a neighbour found my mother face down on the floor in the porch at the front of the house. She didn't know how long Mammy had been there or the circumstances of her being on the floor. Mammy was rushed to the Westshore Hospital emergency room and I received a call in Toronto. It was late August 2012, and I'd recently started a new job. Luckily my boss at the time was understanding and allowed me to go home to attend to my mother. I looked for a flight out to Port-of-Spain two days later. Prior to leaving I searched online for information on seniors' homes in Trinidad and also called on friends to get recommendations.

I rushed to the hospital shortly after landing in the airport. There lay my mother on the bed with drips on her arm. She looked plump and a bit disoriented lying on the bed. Her eyes were wide open and she seemed alert. I gave her a big hug and kiss and asked her if she was fine. She said she was great and wondered when she was going home. The doctor suggested keeping her one more day for observation. In the meantime, we were grappling with the thought of again leaving her alone in her home. It was an undesirable option and the next time she may not be lucky to be discovered by the neighbour. She was forgetful at that stage, but still cognisant of everything that was happening.

Colette, Brent and I decided it was time for her to get 24-hour supervision and be admitted to a seniors' home. This was against her wishes. She had told me many years before that she never wanted to be admitted to 'one of those places'. She felt guilty when her own mother suffering from Alzheimer's disease, died only a few weeks after being admitted to a facility. She had told me then, she would commit suicide if I ever admitted her to a home.

I felt really sad and helpless having to do this, but none of us felt we had the means, skill, or time to take care of our mother and it was the best option. Her pension from working as a teacher in the public school system covered the majority of the monthly fee to stay in a home and we could supplement the rest.

The big question was which facility would be considered

suitable. We had heard one horror story after the next about badly run seniors' home throughout the country.

People would say, 'Every Tom, Dick and Harry is opening an 'Old folks' home' these days. All they want is the money!'

It was a frightening prospect to put one's parent in the hands of total strangers and walk away with the hope that they would do what they said. I asked many friends for recommendations and we visited four or five places. One home was packed with elderly patients staring at a television set in one room and on another porch they stared into space. One woman was tied to a chair, a sad and disturbing scene. Another in a private room called out to everyone passing, 'Hello, Hello'. The nurse smiled and said we needn't bother with her because she called out to people all day. The room available for our mother was a dark interior room with no windows. She said they used to have birthday parties and activities for the elderly, but the owner put them on a tight budget and cut out all the activities. Brent and I walked out of the place feeling like we were looking at death in the face. The people looked drugged and waiting to die.

A seniors' home in St Anne's was said to be run by a 'fancy nurse who lived abroad'. Even though the fees were well out of our means, we visited out of curiosity. People said the home provided board games and activities to stimulate the minds of the residents. The proposed programs were the typical ones one would hear about in North American facilities and not rocket science, except that nobody cared to do more than feed, wash and house the elderly at the majority of local places.

We settled for a home where my high school friend's mother had spent her last days. The facility was a big house within easy reach of the Churchill Roosevelt Highway. My mother would have to share a room with one other person. Even though the rooms were small, I didn't think this was a problem. It would certainly be an advantage if she could speak to another resident. She had spent too many years alone and this may have hastened her dementia. We heard stories that 'good families' put their parents in that home. It might also mean the price was going to be steep. Well, if it was good for the 'special families', then we would have to get our mother a spot. The elitist Trinidadian attitude was always at work with social class influencing everyday decisions.

The owner gave us a short tour to see the facility and convinced us it was suitable. They prepared fresh meals from scratch every day. Families could visit daily within specific times. Their staff all had basic training in Geriatric care, and many residents had been with them for a few years. We were satisfied and a space was available, so we decided to grab this before it was gone.

We then had to determine the best way to break the news to my mother that she was not going back to her beloved house with her little dog, Butch. It was not going to be easy. I would just have to drive her to the place, I thought.

I used the list supplied by the owner of the seniors' home to pack clothing, cosmetics and other supplies for life in the home. When we moved her in a wheelchair to the car on August 31, 2012 her feet were swollen and she couldn't walk. Whatever had caused her collapse had also affected her mobility. We hoped this was temporary and she would have the courage to walk again.

She asked repeatedly, 'Ah going home? Ah going home right?'

All I could say, with guilt, was that she was going to a different home. I couldn't look her in the eyes.

When we arrived at the seniors' home, she asked me, 'What place is this?'

She was forgetful, but not stupid.

I told her she was at a nice new home and the nurse would take good care of her. We tried lifting her up a flight of four steps to the bedroom assigned to her. This was extremely difficult since she was quite plump and heavy.

'She will have to lose that weight,' was the first remark by the owner of the home. 'She's too heavy and we won't be able to lift her.

Was this woman going to starve my mother to death? What did she mean by that statement? I was a bit uneasy.

My mother looked at me with very sad and accusing eyes and didn't say anything. Her eyes said the words she wouldn't utter. We were leaving her in a seniors' home; the type of place she hated with all her heart. I was being wicked to her and she wouldn't speak to me.

'Mammy, you're going to be OK,' I said, but she wouldn't say a word.

Brent and I spoke to her and hugged her for a while and then left. I felt so guilty but it seemed like the best option at the time. We visited the next day and my friend, Lucia came to give Mammy a manicure and pedicure so she could feel better. The care providers changed her clothes and then let us enter her room. Mammy's feet were still swollen and she couldn't walk. Her knees had lost cartilage according to an X-ray and the doctor was sceptical about whether she would be able to walk properly again.

Her roommate was a short skinny woman with curly hair, a Cocoa Panyol (a person of mixed African and Spanish heritage). Her face had a permanent sneer and the look of mischief, as if she was about to make a sarcastic remark. Another character at the home was Jean who rambled in eloquent English about this and that. Tall, with pale skin and blue eyes, this once important diplomat had been reduced to third stage Alzheimer's disease, and no cure in sight. An elderly skinny man was seen running to the front gates on several occasions. He appeared physically healthy and maintained a smirk on his face. Another woman sported a brown handbag and told me she was heading home. She walked around the yard with the handbag and spoke to anyone who would listen, saying she had been brought there against her wishes, and we were to call her family at a specific telephone number. This was very sad since she knew the number from memory and repeated it to her audience.

One elderly resident seemed to be in good health mentally and physically. She asked us to bring magazines for her to read. She was tired of the material at the home and needed mental stimulation. Some patients walked around and helped with tasks in the kitchen as the chef prepared meals, others sat staring out into their own world. The only constant was the drone of the television set used for 'babysitting' or background noise, it wasn't clear. Not many residents looked at the TV.

I left Mammy with a heavy heart at the end of the week, promising to return for her 80th birthday in a few months. I knew she wasn't happy, but I hoped she would somehow get used to the place and cheer up.

Calling every week to check in eased my guilt and I noticed a gradual acceptance as my mother became used to the staff and her new surroundings. Eventually the swelling in her legs went down and she was able to regain mobility. By mid September, the staff told me Mammy was able to use a walker to go to the shower. She walked, holding on to the railings and was bright and chatty. It was really good news for all of us. When my mother's 80th birthday came, I visited as promised, and we set up her party in the large car port at the seniors' home. A few of her friends and a cousin came to celebrate. We brought birthday cake and snacks for all the residents, but those who were diabetic were not allowed to eat the cake. Jean, who babbled incessantly, almost smashed the cake to bits in an excited moment approaching the table. We had to lead her gently back to her chair as one of the elderly gentlemen rushed for the gates. He had to be guided to sit inside. One had to be constantly vigilant with the elderly.

One year rolled into the next and Mammy was able to regain her charm and good spirits. She still recognised my voice and called me by name when I was on the telephone. I noticed by 2014, however she had slipped into more incoherent conversations based on the terms cbc, schwim and schwam.

I would asked what schwim was and she spelled it clearly for me, ' S , C, H, W, I, M'.

When she was in a good mood, our telephone call would be filled with schwims and schwams. Nobody knew where she got these letters from. They could have been a brand name on some device, but they were stuck in her head. During my visit to Trinidad in November 2014 we had an outing to a Parang Festival where groups of singers performed Christmas music sung in Spanish. Mammy was able to walk slowly but surely from the car to the venue. Once she arrived however, she wanted to sit until the end and never wanted to rise, not even to go to the bathroom. I accepted her limitation with concern since we were there for quite a few hours. She ate everything heartily. There was never a problem with her appetite. Even old Parang celebrities were in the audience, albeit a shadow of themselves, suffering from some sort of dementia. Where had all the time gone and why did many of the elders have to age in this way? These were questions that tugged at my brain.

Mammy would sometimes leave the seniors' home to spend a weekend at her own house, or at Brent's house. On one such occasion when I was back in Trinidad for a visit, I had the opportunity to take care of her for a weekend. I made sure she ate all her food at mealtimes and also gave her a shower in the morning.

That morning as she stepped naked over the threshold of the

shower, hanging on to my arm for fear of falling, Mammy remarked, 'You are like my mother now. You are bathing me.'

I almost burst into tears. She realised her precarious situation and her inability to move around without assistance. That was a moment of clarity when she observed her daughter had become her caregiver and mother figure. She held onto the rack of the sliding door as I soaped her body, and it came crashing down. This made her extremely alarmed so I had to comfort her saying it would be OK. No harm was caused. Then it was a challenge getting her out of the shower and into clean clothes. I certainly appreciated the work being done by all the nurses and helpers at the seniors' home. It was not an easy task taking care of the elderly.

My siblings and I continuously questioned whether this was the future we had to look forward to. I would certainly have to use my remaining conscious time on earth and travel far and wide to see the world before my brain and body were lost.

That Christmas, my sister brought both sons, Amiri and Khadir to Trinidad to see Mammy.

'We're not sure how long she'll live,' Colette said vociferously. 'Come and spend time with your Granny!'

I asked her why she kept calling death on our mother I found it very upsetting. Nobody could predict when an elderly person would die, and it made no sense to judge and determine dates.

I also found it upsetting when well meaning friends would

ask my mother's age then say, 'Well, she's had a long life'.

This enraged me. I wanted her to live forever. How dare they act like God trying to predict her death? That Christmas, my mother spent a few days in her own house, sleeping in her own bed. The day she returned to the seniors' home, she stopped walking. According to Colette, she could feel Mammy's spirits drop when she said it was time to go back to the facility. It was as if she had died inside. My mother never waked after that day.

## Constant Decline

My mother's health deteriorated that year. She was resisting eating and my mother usually ate very well. The staff would not move her from the bed since she could no longer walk and my mother stayed in the same room for months without even going outside for fresh air. In my mind it was worse than prison. The home was not equipped with bed lifts and wheel chairs, and made no effort to accommodate residents with special needs. This was ridiculous for facility caring for the elderly. There were flights of steps to enter one level with bedrooms. If one couldn't walk up or down, he or she would not have a chance to sit and watch TV with the others or sit out on the porch to look at the garden.

I became increasing dissatisfied with the service at the home. Colette witnessed one worker being verbally abusive to an elderly gentleman when he complained about being hungry. The residents always complained about being hungry, yet we would see the cook preparing meals in the kitchen every day. Who was getting this food then? Was it never enough?

Colette had sneaked in rotis and pies on a few occasions to feed Mammy and some of her close friends without letting the staff know.

'Forget the diabetes!' She said. 'Let them enjoy themselves once in a while.'

Colette and I overheard the owner of the home saying, if the patient doesn't eat, just give her a liquid supplement.

One occasion when I visited, I was shocked to see all my mother's hair had been cut right down to the scalp. She looked at her reflection in a mirror, lamenting the fact that she used to be beautiful and she'd become ugly. My mother had beautiful hair and it was a shame it was removed without any consultation. When I confronted the owner of the home, she said the family agreed to this.

I screamed at her, 'Who is THE FAMILY? I would never agree to that and my sister lives in the US and would never agree to it either. You've only done this out of convenience so you don't have to comb the patient's hair.'

Thus I accused her and felt it was my right to do so. The less work they had, the better. They knew that my sister and I lived abroad and there was no telling when we would show up in Trinidad, so they could do anything. In addition, my brother was very quiet and more accepting. He wouldn't protest.

I scolded, 'Even if a patient is senile, there's no reason to take advantage of them and disfigure the person like that!'

She didn't like to hear the word 'senile'. I'd seen

documentaries about staff in health care facilities treating the elderly badly, especially when the family was not playing an active part in their care. I was suspicious that the same was happening at the home.

Relocation Again

Colette subsequently moved back to Trinidad in another attempt at settling home. Since our mother was in a facility and the family home lay idle, Colette moved in. Her life in Atlanta was not going well since she left the first time and she couldn't regain a position like her first job. Colette shipped all her belongings to the family home in Diego Martin and did major renovations on the home. She also had a brand new engine installed into my mother's old car to get it running efficiently on the road. She then settled into a routine job in education and would visit my mother at the senior's home weekly to see how she was doing. It was a great relief for me to know two siblings were in Trinidad to keep an eye on Mammy.

They provided continuous updates – 'Gloria ate well this week. She seems to be settling well at the home'.

My mother may not have recognised Colette when she went to visit, but she certainly remembered her car.

'That's my car you know,' she would tell Colette.

## CHAPTER 6

## SALT AND FRESH!

Dry as a Biscuit

I returned home to visit my family after Easter. My sister, Colette and I went to see Mammy at the seniors' home. She looked very ill and sat on a chair motionless. She couldn't move her legs and the attendants complained that she hadn't been eating regularly. In fact, she barely touched her lunch that day when I tried to feed her. I left the place with grave concern and promised to check in the following Monday to see how she was doing. That weekend I had packed many activities into two days and looked forward to an eventful vacation.

I was launching my new publications in Trinidad for the first time and managed to schedule an interview on the Morning Show at CNC3 in Port-of-Spain. The main goal of the interview was to promote my upcoming book launch on the Sunday afternoon. I babbled more than the host of the show, hogging more than my seven minute time slot. I always got carried away when sitting in front of a camera. Friends saw the television interview and sent messages congratulating me on a job well done.

I planned a book launch at the meeting rooms at Alliance Française in Woodbrook on Sunday afternoon and could barely sleep the night before in anticipation of the event. I practiced my speech and book readings a few times to be sure I was ready. The time went quickly. Before I knew it, we had to dress and get to the venue. I had hoped to bring my mother to the event so she would feel proud of me. However, judging from her poor state of health, I had to abandon that idea. It was the first time my whole family helped me with a launch. The most special of all was that my nephews acted as the ushers and took photographs. Colette and my sister-in-law set up the refreshments table and Brent managed book sales. I was also excited to see how many old school friends supported me and came to the event buying my new books. It was a joyful and successful afternoon. After the pressure of the launch was over, I was finally able to relax and get some sleep.

Early Monday morning, Brent received a call from the Rion home. The nurse said Mammy hadn't eaten anything all weekend and we should take her to the hospital. It sounded urgent, so we got dressed and went directly to the home. I'd taken some ripe papaya to try feeding her when I got there. She really looked feeble and wretched lying on her bed and could barely open her eyes. I asked one of the attendants to cut up the papaya and bring it to me so I could feed her. She cut it into large pieces which were placed on a dish. I crushed the papaya into pulp and tried to feed Mammy, giving her small morsels to swallow. She ate a few bits slowly as I coaxed and encouraged.

'Yummy, yummy. It's so good for you,' I said as I forced her to eat, trying to hold back the tears.

She smiled ever so slightly revealing one upper tooth. Her plate of false teeth had been removed in case she choked on it at night. I saw one of the attendants come around to watch, as if doubting that I could get my mother to eat. With a lot of persuasion, she accepted some of the fruit.

We called for an ambulance to take her to a nearby private hospital. The emergency ambulance staff lifted my mother, her sheets, pillow, and all onto a stretcher to make it easier to take her off the bed. My mother screamed in pain and fear. She was strapped to the stretcher and then wheeled to the ambulance and loaded in through the back door. I travelled with her in the vehicle to the hospital to try and comfort her along the way. When we arrived at the private hospital, we were taken to a triage room where a nurse took her vital signs. Brent was directed to the cashier to pay an instalment. The emergency room was pristine and the floors shone. No patients were visible in any other rooms and the area was relatively quiet. A physician came right away to do an assessment. He asked my mother her name and I was surprised when she answered promptly, 'Gloria James.' I was so impressed that she could say her name while she was obviously in a great deal of pain. Her blood pressure was dangerously low and so was her heart rate. She was admitted into the intensive care unit (ICU).

After an hour or so, the senior doctor called us into ICU. He spoke in a very caring tone. 'You can come and speak to your mother for a short time and then we have to leave her to rest,' he said. We went in to see her hooked up to many tubes and instruments. Her heart rate and blood pressure flashed on a screen. Everything looked too low for comfort. She was receiving oxygen through a mask on her face and wires were attached to her chest. She was also being fed saline solution through an intravenous tube that entered a vein in her hand. When we said hello, she tried to answer but then slumped into sleep. We were then ushered out of the room to get a synopsis of the situation.

'Your mother is gravely ill,' said the doctor. 'She's as dry as a biscuit!' he said.

'What do you mean by that?' I asked.

The doctor explained his care plan and explained his findings up to that time. Mammy was so dehydrated, it seemed that she hadn't received water for a long time and all the electrolytes in her blood were out of balance.

The second day we went to visit, her condition was improving slightly and the nurse said she was able to feed her a light soup. This was encouraging, but all the electrolytes still needed stabilizing and her blood sugar level was still too high. As we paid the second day's bills and looked at the estimate for day three, Colette said we were crazy to continue with the private hospital.

'We will be bankrupt soon and won't even be able to pay for a funeral if she were to die. We need to take Mammy to a public hospital!'

'No, No!' Brent and I protested. 'We don't trust the public hospitals,' we said.

'Well, you'll regret it when you can't pay the bills here!' she said.

After going through all the unpaid expenses and those that would be owed on the third day, it totalled at least $30,000.00. We decided we would surely have to take our chances at a public hospital, but it was one of our greatest fears. We reserved an ambulance to take Mammy across to a nearby public hospital.

On entering the emergency ward, I realised the situation was very different to the calm and pristine private hospital we had just left. The casualty ward looked like a war zone. We could not even get a stretcher for Mammy because they were all occupied. Capacity was so high that patients were being treated on stretchers in the hallways. No beds were available on any of the wards. We all stood with our mother observing the scene as doctors ran in many directions and nurses of all shapes and sizes also ran around: locals, Filipinos, Africans, Indians, Syrians, and Cubans. I was surprised by the ethnic diversity of the work force. I had not seen such diversity when I left the country twenty years before. No one person seemed to be in charge and nobody made eye contact. I wondered if anyone would ever come to my mother's attention. After almost two hours, a stretcher became available.
A stout, young female doctor came with a chart to ask about

my mother's condition. I told her as much as I knew and gave her referral documents and test results from the private hospital. She took notes then disappeared. Colette, Brent and I took turns in standing next to my mother, while alternating taking a seat in the waiting area outside. A man sat in a wheelchair with his faithful wife, who was standing behind him for hours. They faced the direction of the medical station, with the doctors and nurses who seemed pre-occupied, writing copious notes about various patients. They never looked up.

The wife said, 'All we need are the X-ray results. Hello, hello. Somebody? Anybody? Doctor, doctor…' she tried to stop a small Cuban man with glasses and a stethoscope who was running past.

'I am not the doctor,' he said with a heavy accent. 'I am the nurse.'

He continued running and later came and gave my mother an injection on her skin to test for irritation and an allergic reaction. 'Ask her if it's itching her,' he said.

'She really can't speak for herself at this time,' I tried to explain.

He ran along on his way without listening and came back in ten minutes looking for bumps or sign of a rash. He then promptly administered some medication.

'What is this? What are you giving her?' I asked.

He didn't answer and continued running on to the next patient.

After five hours, a massive change of staff occurred as the evening shift came in. A new young doctor came to ask me the same questions I had answered before about my mother. I went through everything I knew and he took notes. I also told him she did not get anything to eat. He said nobody would have time to feed her so she would need a feeding tube, and he was gone, never to be seen again. Late that night, we left our names with a customer representative at a nearby desk informing her that our mother could not speak for herself and we would return later that night to follow up. We left our mother on a stretcher in the corridor of a crazy emergency ward. Guilt was killing us to leave her side and since we could barely sleep, we returned to the hospital at midnight to assess the situation. When we got there, no doctors were around and the area was quiet. I saw the same middle aged man sitting on the wheel chair, facing the direction of the medical station, still waiting for his X-ray.

One Filipina nurse was doing the rounds and checking equipment. We saw her rolling Mammy into one of the side rooms. After ten hours, a spot finally became available in a side room off the emergency area, but still, this was not on a ward. I tried asking this nurse many questions about what had happened. She didn't know anything because she had just started her shift. I asked if my mother was given anything to eat. She eventually went to the chart and saw that a doctor had tried to put a feeding tube down my mother's throat, but she bit him. I almost laughed out loud. This must have been a wicked and painful procedure and Mammy responded accordingly by biting the perpetrator. She was ill, but still feisty. We decided there and then to get her discharged and moved to the public hospital in Port-of-Spain the next day.

The following morning we came early and asked to have her discharged. After a few hours of spinning and posturing with hospital staff we were finally able to get one of the young doctors to discharge Mammy. With that, we took off for the public hospital in Port-of-Spain in an ambulance hired for the next transfer. We sped down the Priority Bus Route and as we entered downtown Port-of-Spain, the driver turned on the siren at full blast. I felt a bit important as we made our way swiftly to the hospital and traffic cleared a way for us to pass.

'Do you hear the siren Mammy?' I asked, as I sat in the back holding her hand and comforting her. 'It's all for you. You're going to get better!'

Fortunately, traffic wasn't bad since most people were leaving downtown during rush hour and we were heading in the opposite direction into town. We were off to a new adventure at another hospital.

It Will Happen But When?

In what seemed like record time, we entered the front of the emergency ward at the hospital and as we entered with the stretcher, the security guard announced we were at the wrong entrance. That was actually the entrance for pedestrians and the stretcher barely made it around the bend, but then we were fine. I thanked the driver and attendant profusely and my mother was sent directly to a triage booth. There was no need to wait for a stretcher or any unnecessary delays. Countless stretchers and wheel chairs were readily available. It was Thursday night and a crowd was in the waiting room outside. However, there seemed to be order and a system was in place. The area was relatively clean and all the nurses wore crisp uniforms. It was definitely a different atmosphere to the one we left at the hospital in the East.

A nurse took my mother's vital signs and asked me questions. I was then asked to sit at the side until called again. The security at this hospital was very strict, only letting in one family member per patient. There was no bending of the rules, so Colette sat outside with other family members. A young female doctor came to ask questions about my mother's health. Her questions seemed a bit strange and I had to correct her on a few occasions.

'Didn't she come from the St. James Medical Clinic?' the

doctor asked.

'No she's was actually at the hospital in the East,' I said. After a while, I realised the doctor was asking me questions from the wrong patient's chart in her hand. She was enquiring about Mrs. Anthony! I wondered if this was a sign of the healthcare to come. I breathed in and out and tried to maintain my composure. Then, two young doctors came to ask a host of questions and take notes. I knew it was a teaching hospital but the medical staff looked very young. Or maybe I was getting old and young professionals looked like they could be my children! I gave them the referrals from the private hospital and explained every detail I knew about my mother's condition and her treatment to date. The lead doctor took copious notes while the other just looked on. He asked more and more questions and took notes. He then asked me to sit outside again until called. The air-conditioning unit was cranked up to full power and the room was extra cold in this area.

I had to go outside for a little air and something to eat before I became ill. I asked the security woman to take a good look at my face since I was coming out only for a short while and would want to re-enter.

'Why are you coming out?' she asked. 'Well I have to eat before I collapse and become another patient in emergency.' With that I was out. A strange and erratic man walked around the visitors' waiting room with a clip board pretending to take names and count fares for a vehicle. The television in the waiting room was running, but he provided much needed entertainment for family members during the many hours of waiting. Colette and I went to a fast food place opposite for fried chicken, ate hastily and then returned to the entrance to the emergency ward. The security guards had changed shift and the person in charge didn't know us. This was beneficial, because we could do our own changing of the guards. I asked Colette to go in with the bags of clothes and I would stay outside and wait. After spending a total of five hours, in the casualty section the staff found a bed for my mother on ward 34. Colette called on her cell phone with the joyful news from the ward. It was 11:00 pm and Brent had arrived at the hospital by that time. We managed to sneak around a back way and up some steps to the ward on the third floor while a security guard took a nap on the bench nearby. We wanted to see Mammy settle in her bed. The nurse on duty seemed fairly pleasant and she had an accent from another Caribbean country. Her pleasant demeanour put me at ease. She said, however, that my mother scratched her while she was trying to dress her. I apologized profusely for my mother's bad behaviour and then looked at her and said, 'Mammy be nice to the nurse now. She'll take good care of you.' My mother smiled innocently like a small child and sent me a kiss. Then she sent a kiss in the air for the nurse as well. My siblings and I were anxious to return next morning to meet the doctors and learn more about her condition.

Ward 34

The following morning we arrived early to witness what I called the Elaborate 19th Century Protocol and Dance of Doctors and Nurses. The buildings looked dated from the 1940's. Boxes of paper records could be seen near the entrance to the wards. Even though the beds were from this century, they did not match the dated building. The nurses didn't readily provide information about the patient's treatment and older nurses completely ignored family members if questions were asked. Some young nurses were friendly and would speak to people directly and maybe give information about the patient's care. Doctors passed once a day during the morning on the wards.

We were fortunate that visiting hours had recently changed to 7:00 am - 9:30 am instead of 11:00 am - 12:30 pm or else we would never have met the doctors. When they spoke, they seldom gave details about the patients' care plan, and seldom give details to family members, especially if one was too quiet and not knowledgeable about healthcare. In noticing the arrogance, I was determined to beat them at their game. After all, I had every right to know what drugs they were feeding my mother. I wanted to look up the side effects and challenge the care if it didn't make sense to me. I was a fussy family member, and I knew it.

I asked a hundred questions of the main doctor in the group who did the rounds looking at my mother that morning. I wanted him to speak to me. By my fourth question he seemed a little irritated.

'Anything else?' he asked.

'Yes, what is that big bump on the back of her neck? Is that a swollen lymph node? Have you seen it?' I asked.

Even if he hadn't noticed this, he said he did just to be nice, and told me it was not a swollen lymph node. The doctors and nurses might have missed this. I only found the huge golf ball-sized bump when I was adjusting Mammy's pillow. Proper bedside manners were obviously not on the nursing or medical school curriculum. If good customer service wasn't an inherent personality, then patients and families received the brunt of whatever frustration the staff member was facing. The saga continued as Mammy was being treated for a host of ailments with no simple solution: antibiotics for an infection which looked like it had spread to the blood, insulin for high blood sugar, a constant saline drip to re-hydrate the body. Her left leg was swollen to twice the size of the other leg and the doctor said she may have a blood clot. They had to take an ultra-sound of her leg. This test was ordered but we had to wait a few days before she was taken to the clinic for examination.

She wasn't alert during the evening visits and would frequently dose off. However in the morning visiting hours, she seemed more alert and ready to communicate. I asked the doctor what they planned to feed her since on the first day I saw the tea lady drop off a big sandwich and a cup of tea to her bedside. I had to tell the woman that my mother was too weak to lift a cup and certainly wouldn't be able to hold a piece of bread and bring it to her mouth, far less chew the bread. However, she still needed to be fed something. By the second day in the hospital, we finally got this fact clear; she needed liquid food. We were realizing how involved we had to be in our mother's healthcare for things to progress smoothly. I planned to be at her beside everyday during the morning and evening visiting times. It was like a job. I also decided to make my own smoothies with raw vegetables and fresh fruits, and take these to her so she could get something fresh into her system.

Colette and I observed all the patients on this side of Ward 34 trying to guess their ailments and we made friends with their family and guests. An elderly woman with cancer was on the bed opposite and her daughter came to make her comfortable everyday. Another Granny to the left of her told all the nurses she was 94 and needed a cup of tea.
'I'm awake so long and can't get a cup of tea,' she complained.
One woman near the window asked me to help her get a drink of water. 'I have my bottle,' she said.

I felt sorry for the poor woman in the sweltering afternoon heat. No nurses paid her any attention and the heat was unbearable. I poured some water from the bottle into her mouth and squirmed as I saw her three rotten teeth. She swallowed greedily. The poor wretch was thirsty.
The young woman in the bed next to Mammy became our spy and we even gave her a telephone number to contact us in case something was to happen to our mother.
One morning she said she overheard the doctors saying, 'Things don't look too good. You have to tell the family.'

Another morning she overheard one doctor say, 'Her
recovery is remarkable. She's doing so well.'

We were lucky to have our spy until the day she was
discharged from the hospital. I was happy for this young
woman whose husband and siblings came to visit her and
bring food every day. She was too young to be in this ward
with elderly patients.

During the evenings visiting hours, evangelical people
walked around the wards praying for patients if the families
wanted prayers. I asked them to come to pray for Mammy.
Any prayers would be good at that stage.

'Jesus bless yuh sistah!' said one.

'Yes Lord,' said the other.

She had a bible in the air and dramatically continued her
prayer with eyes closed.

'Pray for your sistah I beg you Lord. Sistah Gloria needs
your help.' With that Mammy looked at them and smiled.
After a few more phrases of praise, we thanked them and
they packed up and moved to the bed of the 94 years old
woman. While they prayed for her, she spoke non-stop, not
hearing a word they were saying.

'I am 94 years old you know. I don't know why they brought
me to the hospital. If only I could get a cup ah tea,' the old
woman said. 'Call the nurse to bring ah cup of tea for mih.'

We laughed as the cutest Granny focused on her tea and
didn't even hear the prayers. After a while, the God-fearing
pair packed up and moved on to their next willing recipient
of prayers.

When we left the hospital that evening, we drove through St.
James and I anxiously searched the store fronts for a fan to
put at my mother's bedside. The ward was not cooled with
air-conditioning and the temperature could reach 34 degrees
in the shade. She needed a fan to keep air moving and create
some relief from the heat. Since nobody was around to give
her water from the bottle we left at her bedside during the

day, a good fan was critical. At a hardware store, I saw a sign for floor fans being sold at $99. We pulled aside right away to grab this special deal. As I bought the fan I felt dizzy with the heat. All I saw on the front of the fan was a cartoon of a donkey. The attendant plugged it in to ensure that it worked.

'This fan comes with a one day warranty,' he said smiling.

'What do you mean a one day warranty? Is the fan any good or will it break down the minute I walk out yuh store?' I asked.

He and the cashier laughed heartily. He said, 'I meant to say 24 hours guarantee!' and we all laughed heartily.
I hoped the flimsy fan would hold up to the ravages of the hospital. All we had to do was plug it in and leave it on day and night. On a few occasions when we visited the ward, we found the fan pushed to a corner, and switched off with the top on the floor. This could have happened when Mammy was taken for lab tests or she was turned from one side to the next by hospital staff. She was supposed to be turned periodically to help heal the bed sores. Some tight-fitting compression stockings were placed on her legs to prevent blood clots. The stocking left a huge dent mid-thigh in the swollen leg and it looked extremely painful to me. When I asked one doctor about this, he said it was supposed to fit tight, but I had my doubts. When some friends visited my mother during her second week in the hospital, I noticed the brand name of the fan was 'Bad Ass'. How could I have bought a product with that brand name? That explained the cartoon of the donkey and probably explained the laughter when I purchased the gadget.

Cleaning staff mopped the floors but ignored the ledges. We saw the dust of years on all shelves. In fact the dust and termite hills had a firm residence in the shelves next to my mother's bed. The fans were also caked in dust and the occasional bird flew through the windows and into the ward at will, sometimes resting on ledges. If one was not careful, a bird could peck at breakfast! The first week at the ward turned into a second week and I extended my stay another week before returning to Toronto. I had to see some sort of stability in my mother's condition before I could feel comfortable returning to a home thousands of miles away. I also wanted to find a new seniors' home because I was not satisfied with the care at the first place. We wanted to find a place where she could rest comfortably after being discharged from the hospital.

Quito-quito

With only a few days remaining of my visit to Trinidad I started a quest to find the 'ideal' new senior's home as quickly as possible. The search became frantic as I combed the internet and found a list of many registered seniors' homes around the country. The challenge was then to find a reasonably priced place which offered the best service, and was within driving distance from my siblings in the northwest region of the country. I made a list of places and phone numbers and called a few friends to see if they had recommendations. Nobody seemed to want to give firm advice about any one place. They had heard unsavoury rumours about many facilities. I then decided to call those within driving distance to find out if they had vacancies. Only then could Brent and I drive around to each place for a visit. The first two I called had no vacancy, and I was starting to panic. What if I didn't find a place? What if the doctors decided to discharge Mammy in a few days time? What were we going to do? I then called another place which was near our neighbourhood. They had a huge fee but they had a vacancy. I outlined my long list of requirements to the nurse in charge as I spoke to her on the telephone and wondered if she was laughing at me in the background. At any rate, I made an appointment for the next day to see the facility.

After making that appointment, I called a neighbour who was a retired nurse and asked her about the place. She reminded me it was the small facility where my ailing Granny had gone many years ago, and died just a few days after. I had forgotten about them, and swiftly changed my mind. They had a big price but bad reputation. I continued combing the internet and spotted a website for a new senior's home, Burt's Manor, in the mountains of the Northern Range. The facility was advertised well online and looked like a beautiful guest house and spa. I wondered how this could be a home for the aged. It was a bit off the beaten path. However, I reasoned if Mammy were to stay in the mountains, she'd have clean fresh air to breathe everyday and the area would be calm and restful. It would be the best place to recover from illness and pass the time. I called the owner for information and then made an appointment to visit the next day.

When I told my siblings about the Manor in the mountains, they were a bit apprehensive.

'Why does she have to go so far? Dat place is behind God back. It's in quito-quito (a slang describing a remote location). Nobody would be going to visit her quite to hell up there!' was the response I got.

'I don't care,' I said. 'If it offers the services we're looking for, then we'll reserve her spot.'

Brent and I went to visit the next day and found the place to be very spacious and comfortable. The staff seemed friendly, qualified and well organised. We were even greeted by the dog, Captain, a friendly pit bull dog who came to say hello when we walked in. A sprinkling of residents sat in the porch and in the living-room and the owner did a wonderful job of describing his qualifications and his future plans for the home. I was immediately impressed and asked him to save a place for Mammy when she would be discharged from the hospital. We made a swift decision just based on gut feelings about the place.

Days at the Ward

'It's the nuts man. Salt and Fresh! Cashew nuts, kumar, rice cake!'

'Salt and Fresh! Cashew nuts, kumar, rice cake!'

The roadway exiting the hospital was filled with vendors who plied their trade as hospital staff and visitors entered and left everyday. Some vendors paid for space in a wooden building where they sold all manner of snack food and drinks. Others would set up a makeshift table at the side of the pavement and take a chance, especially targeting families as they came and went during visiting hours.

There was the nuts man who sat with his tray of miscellaneous plastic bags filled with goodies. The doubles man and the pie man attracted a line of customers early in the morning, as people entered the hospital grounds and needed breakfast. I was a bit sceptical about buying food from these people who handled food and money with great dexterity. No hand washing facilities were visible for miles around.

The herbs man pulled up in a pick-up truck, opened the tray and called on departing hospital staff, as well as the hundreds of families on their way out at 6:00 pm. His spoken English was impeccable compared to that of the other vendors who spoke in broken English. He explained the virtues of his herbs to anyone who would listen. Small plants were ready for transplanting in the garden or could be harvested fresh from the window sill in your kitchen daily. A woman sold slices of cake from a tray on the edge of the car park: sponge cake, black fruit cake, lemon cake. They were large tempting slices for anyone who felt hungry on the way out.

The parking lot security staff were a strange breed. It was their job to make the free parking lot at the hospital as difficult as possible for all visitors. The lot was open early in the morning and cones were placed in some of the best and most convenient spots along the edge of the parking lot so nobody could use those spots. Only when the worst spots were filled would they begrudgingly move the cones. This caused great frustration and ire in many visitors. The side for staff parking seldom filled up, but one was not allowed to park on that side of the parking lot unless you could somehow make friends with the attendant. The parking staff all went home at 6:00 pm sharp, locking the gate to exit the visitors' parking lot onto a nearby street. This time coincided with the end of visiting hours when a mass exodus from the hospital entered their cars to leave, creating long lines of traffic. We all tried to exit through a narrow roadway around buildings to another side of the hospital. The gate closure at 6:00 pm defied logic.

One morning a frustrated relative who had parked on the street walked through the parking lot at the end of visiting hours and saw the cones still fixed in spaces near the edge of the parking lot. She decided to challenge the bossy looking attendant for not allowing people to park in the space. Suddenly a huge argument broke out and it turned ugly.

'Why all yuh so stupid? You have the cones in the space and people have to park outside,' she said.

'Ma'am, mind yuh business and keep walking,' said the

111

attendant.

Well, that comment really irritated the woman who decided to spend another ten minutes berating the parking lot attendant.

'That is why you still working in a parking lot. You're uneducated and it's the only job you could get!' said the irate visitor.

'Ma'am, ah said to mind yuh business! I'm in charge of this parking lot,' said the attendant.

'What de hell? Ah sure you don't even own a car! Yuh too blasted stupid. Why de hell you don' give people a space to park? I have to walk quite to hell outside and you hogging up all the spaces in here!'

This visitor was fuming. The women argued back and forth and it seemed like a fist fight could break out at any moment. The visitor was not backing down. I asked Colette to drive out quickly so we wouldn't get caught in traffic leaving the site because of a fight. The sun was beating down on us and the morning dew had long burned off.

We were trying to back out of the space as some more people were entering and leaving the parking lot. As we backed out slowly, we barely missed an elderly woman with a short white afro who walked through the parking lot. She was dressed in a pink cotton night gown on her way somewhere. She walked with purpose and in my assessment could not have been very ill. However, she sported her hospital tag on her wrist and was apparently a patient. The old woman decided to walk directly behind our car as we tried to leave. We were to see her at 9:00 am sharp every morning as we left the parking lot that week. She was a hospital regular.

A week after my mother was admitted to the hospital, I saw a nurse ceremoniously approach with a name tag and place it on my mother's wrist. I couldn't believe that after a full week of occupying a bed on the ward and being taken to the X-ray lab and other locations in the hospital, she was only then getting a name tag! Suppose she was left by an attendant on her stretcher in the wrong X-ray room. Nobody would've known who she was. Suppose… Suppose… She could have been Jane Doe in the hospital. She couldn't speak for herself and only on a good day, by some miracle, would she state her name emphatically, then dose off. I didn't know whether to laugh or cry. Progress was being made at the hospital, but one couldn't rush the staff.

'It will happen, but when?' became our mantra.

This same week we noticed an X-Ray film tucked neatly in the corner at the foot of her bed. However on examining the large envelope, I also noticed another large envelope tucked into the foot of the bed. It had the name, 'Mister Maharaj' neatly printed at the front. Brent and I looked at the envelope in shock and hoped that no diagnosis was being made on our mother related to the chest X-ray results of Mr. Maharaj. This was the classic joke of the day for us. I calmly took the envelope and presented it to the nurse at the nurses' station.

'There must be some mistake here,' I said. 'The wrong X-ray film was on my mother's bed.'

She opened her eyes, made no response and calmly put the envelope next to the many stacks of papers which they seemed intent on filling out by hand, day after day. I wished the wards would get computers and enter the 21st century. They were drowning in papers and folders for their patients and I questioned how anyone could keep track of records effectively.

## Maybe on Monday

My mother's youngest sister, Audrey was retired and lived in Florida, and she decided to come to see her sick sister. When she arrived, we drove directly to the hospital to get there in time for the evening visiting hours. She said prayers and wept creating great drama.

I told Mammy, 'There's your sister Audrey. Do you see her?' I said this a few times.

Then suddenly, out of nowhere, my mother said, 'Hi Audrey.'

We didn't expect this. It was a miracle and we all screamed. She had spoken, and made sense. Somewhere behind all the illness and dementia, a few moments of clarity existed. It was a momentous occasion during her stay at the hospital.

One day when we visited, we noticed one of my mother's arms had been tied to the bed railing to prevent her from taking out the drips. Poor Mammy; even when they removed the drips her hand was still tied. We had to release her. It seemed like a cruel act even if it was to prevent mischief. My last day in town was approaching and I wanted to be sure to have the opportunity to speak to a doctor about my mother's condition. The visiting hours had been changed back to lunch time and doctors only made their rounds in the morning around 9:00 am. What a dilemma it was for me. How was I going to be able to speak to them if they were not around during visitation at lunch? I was prepared to stalk them around the hospital to see when they went to lunch.

The night before leaving the ward, I approached nurses at the station to let them know I was flying back to Canada. I wanted to speak to a doctor about my mother's treatment before I left. I asked the whole group loudly at the station what I should do; after all, the doctors only came in the morning to visit the patients. They all stared at me in silence. I might as well have been speaking to myself. The numbness of their reaction was baffling. After a few loud seconds of silence, a sympathetic Cuban nurse looked at me and said in her best English, 'You go to the security on de Charlotte Street and ask for a pass.'

'What security? Where should I go?' I asked.

She explained again, 'The security near the gate will give you a pass to get in early.'

Well thank goodness someone had a conscience. So it was possible to fly past the security at the foot of the elevator after all. Why couldn't the local nurses tell me the same thing? Why did they guard this secret so carefully? She could have seen my distress in having to leave the country with my mother being so ill. As we left the hospital that night, I saw the same Cuban nurse and she pointed at the security booth where I was to get the pass. I thanked her and ran across to speak to the young woman in the booth.

'Hello, I'm leaving the country this weekend and I need to come into the hospital early in the morning to speak to the doctors about my mother's care. What should I do?'

She just stared at me and said nothing.

'Is this where I have to pick up a pass to get in the ward early in the morning?'

Again there was no response. I felt as if I was speaking to a wall, as she tried to formulate what answer to give me.

'Will you give me a pass now?' I continued, not backing down since I knew she was the all important gate keeper, similar to the parking lot attendants.

'When you come in the morning you will get a pass.' Finally she was able to speak to me after observing me from head to toe and letting me babble on!

'Well thanks so much! I'll be here in the morning,' I said, and ran off to the parking lot wondering what power struggle was happening in her mind.

The next morning I was there bright and early at 8:00 am in front of the booth. Miraculously, it was the same young woman.

'Hello I would like a pass to get into Ward 34 please.'

Without saying a word, she stamped a date on a little piece of paper, signed it and gave it to me. Was that what a pass looked like? I was expecting something more official. However, I was thankful for the 'free ticket' and went on my way. I presented my pass to the security guards who manned the elevators up to the ward.

'I have a pass to get in early,' I said.

A security guard took the paper from me and said I could go ahead. This meant I could not come back around. If I left I had no pass to show again. I went directly to the ward, walked past the nurses' station and went straight to my mother's bedside. After a few minutes the nurse in charge came around and asked what I was doing there. I told her I was there to speak with a doctor about my mother's care.

'You can't just walk in here and sit down. This is not the time for visitors!' she said.

'Well I told all the nurses last night that I was coming early in the morning to speak with a doctor because I'm leaving the country.'

'Go in the waiting room and stay over there. I'll call you when the doctors come,' she said. 'You should have taken care of that before since you knew you were leaving the country.'

The rude woman was taking a stab at me because she could do it. The waiting room was around a blind corner and I knew I'd never see when the doctors zipped by to do their three-minute assessment of patients. I decide to pace the floor. I could never stay in the waiting area. I wandered near the pantry and then asked one of the student doctors if she knew when the other doctors were coming around. She had no clue and only focused on her own patients. Everyone was assigned to specific patients. The evil nurse saw me again on the ward and urged me to go back to the waiting area. Never being one to follow instructions, I went out on the balcony and spied on them through the windows waiting to see when the doctors would pass. I decided to stand near the pantry and stake out the people entering and leaving as if I were a sentinel on duty.

Every once in a while, the nurse would pass and look at me. After an hour had passed I saw a noisy group of young doctors passing and sure enough, that particular group had worked with my mother since she was admitted.

'Doctor Clark,' I screamed as the young leader stopped to wash his hands at the hand wash station. I startled him, since no visitors were around at the time. 'I need to speak to you about my mother.'

'Please give me a few minutes to look at the patient and I will be right with you,' he said.

I was lucky I had maintained my post because the nurse in charge certainly had not come to call me. As the rest of his group disappeared, he approached with my mother's chart. I told him I was returning to Canada and needed to know about my mother's progress and treatment to date. I had a list of questions!

'Ms. James she's improved a lot since we admitted her to Ward 34,' he said with a straight face, as he saw my little scrap of paper with questions. 'Do you have questions for me?'

I continued by asking about the blood test results, white blood cell count, her blood sugar levels, the kidney function, the ultrasound results of her leg, a bone cancer test they had said they would do, possible fluid on her lungs, and anything else I could remember. I knew it was the last time they would get a full medical grilling and I had to be the family member to find out the details. He re-assured me they were trying to manage her ailments and she had progressed significantly. Her electrolytes had stabilized and they were monitoring the blood sugar levels.

I looked him in the eyes squarely and said, 'Do your best! She's my mother, so I'm expecting great things from you. Thanks for your help.'

He gave a slight smile and with that he was off. I tried to keep calm so I could leave the hospital without bawling and crying. I was satisfied that progress had been made and held my breath for the remaining time Mammy would spend in the hospital. I hoped and prayed she would be fine.

I prayed that God would bless her with a few caring nurses to help ease her discomfort and aid in her healing. This was a tall order under the circumstances. I planned to return at 4:00 pm for the evening visiting hours and as I left the hospital, I saw the old woman in the pink cotton nightgown walking briskly with a bandaged leg in the direction of the gate. The morning regulars were there too: the nuts man, the doubles man, the pie man, the sauce man and others who frequented the hospital grounds.

Mother's Day was coming up that Sunday and I was to fly out Sunday morning to spend the evening with my daughter in Toronto. I wondered what I could possibly give an ailing mother who dosed off most of the time, and as far as we knew, did not quite understand what was happening around her. I picked some colourful pieces of croton branches from the garden and a few Heliconia flowers, and made a small arrangement from the plants at our family home. The intense dry season had ravaged most of the plants in the garden. It was good to harvest the best of what was left. If nothing else, she could look at the flowers on the ledge near her bed and enjoy them. The floral arrangement would be a distraction from the termite mounds. Close to 4:00 pm, Colette, my aunt and I arrived at the hospital and waited anxiously for the clock to strike 4:00 pm so the important security guards would allow us to use the elevator to the third floor. I knew it was the last time I would be going up to the ward and it was a very emotional time for me.

There was Mammy on her bed sometimes looking around, sometimes nodding off. Her Bad Ass fan was working away to circulate the intensely hot afternoon air. We thought the fan was finally out of commission, but it was re-assembled by one of the staff members. I sang for Mammy, hugged her and she managed to kiss my forehead. I looked at her asked her to promise me that she would get better. I'm not sure if she understood but she certainly nodded at my request.

'You have to get better. That's why you're here. You have to continue to live.' I wept uncontrollably while hugging her.

We noticed that she was no longer wearing the compression stockings. As one of the Cuban nurses passed by taking blood pressure readings, I asked her what had happened to the stockings. She said they got dirty when they were changing Mammy.

'So aren't you going to put on a new pair? Her left leg is still swollen and there's a risk of a blood clot going to the heart. You know that, don't you?'

She replied with a blank face, 'Well the head nurse left with the key for the cupboard, so when she comes on Monday, we will see if there are any stockings in the cupboard.'

I was fuming at that point. How could the head nurse leave the hospital with a key for a cupboard with essential supplies?

'Tell me the name of the stockings so I can go and buy some,' I said.

'They are very expensive,' she said. 'I don't care what they cost! Tell me where I can buy them!' I replied, really losing my patience with this woman.

'I don' ah know where to buy them,' she continued.

'Well tell me the name … What is the Brand name?' My blood was boiling and I felt like strangling her.

'It is Ted,' she said.

'Ted? What is Ted?' I asked.

'The stocking is called Ted,' she continued.

'Well, what size should I get? Small, medium, or large?' I asked.

'I don' ah know. Wait a minute, I check her file,' she said as she went off to look at my mother's records.

Colette suggested I go to the nearest SupFam, a large pharmacy in Maraval to find the stockings. I left immediately since there was no time to lose. Visiting hours ended at 6:00 pm and I didn't want to have to fight off the security at the elevator to get the stockings to my mother. I ran to the parking lot, and drove like a mad woman around the Queens Park Savannah towards Maraval. There was traffic on Maraval Road and I cursed the ever present line of cars in both directions. How was I going to get back on time?

I finally spotted SupFam as I turned a roundabout, and quickly entered the first parking lot on the left. It was the wrong parking lot so I walked across the yard to the store. I walked toward the pharmacists counter looking at the shelves along the way and quickly spotted the TED brand of compression stockings. That was what the nurse was trying to tell me. They were over $200 Trinidad dollars but it didn't matter. One could never put a price on life and death. The dilemma was what size I should buy. I approached one of the helpers at the pharmacist's counter, but she was busy discussing the virtues of a hot sauce with another attendant, and they were too distracted to take notice of me.

'Hello, I'd like some help in deciding what size compression stocking to buy please,' I said.

'Well, what size is the patient?' One girl finally asked.

'She's about my size,' I confirmed. 'Do you have a tape measure?' The dimensions on the box showed calf circumference, distance from the hip to the ankle, thigh circumference, and other dimensions in centimetres. It was a bit tricky so I pulled up my trouser on one side and measured my own leg. In the end, I got a pair of medium stockings and went to the front cashier to check out. It was then a mad dash in the afternoon heat and traffic back to the hospital.

As I parked and arrived at the elevators to the third floor, I had fifteen minutes left. I ran into the ward and Colette and I managed to pull the stockings onto my mother's legs. As the nurse passed, I showed her.

'Look what I bought. It's a medium size and it fit just fine,' I said.

All she did was open her eyes. Before we could say much, the bell rang and visiting hours were over. I hugged my mother and bawled and cried. I didn't know when I'd see her again.

I just put everything in God's hands. Mammy had survived so far and would just have to continue surviving. I had to hang onto Colette for support as I left the ward and entered the elevator for the last time before my flight back to Toronto in the morning.

## CHAPTER 7

## DAYS AT THE MANOR

Mountain Life

After leaving Trinidad, I called daily to find out what was happening with my mother. I pestered my siblings for updates about her progress at the hospital. Finally, after a week and a half, she was discharged from the hospital with her medication. The hospital was generous enough to supply an ambulance to take her to a different seniors' home in St. Joseph. The driver and his attendant did not realise that when Brent told them the place was far, it was really in quito-quito *(a slang describing a remote location)*, in the mountains. As they followed his car through the hills and around blind corners, with a precipice on either side of the road, he could see the ambulance driver in the rear view mirror wincing at every sharp turn in the narrow road. They all hoped no car was coming down the hill in the other direction, or it would have been an elaborate dance to determine who would reverse to a place of safety, for the other to pass.

'Where she staying? Quite up dere? Ah doubt my car could make it up de hill!' was the response of many old friends and neighbours.

My first visit back to Trinidad after Mammy was admitted to the Manor, I travelled on Boxing Day, to benefit from the reduced airline ticket prices and also in time to celebrate her 83rd birthday. I wanted to see my mother's progress and observe if everything was going well at the new home. I wasn't sure if she would recognise me, but this didn't matter. All I wanted to know was that she was receiving the best care possible. The first day I arrived in the country, I rushed to the mountain home to see Mammy. As I entered her room, I held my breath. My mother had lost a lot of weight and she seemed to be half her original size. However, she was able to feed herself slowly, or eat and drink with assistance. I took family albums and a family picture book and read to her. Her smile was infectious that morning and she sent me many kisses in the air. I hugged my mother and rejoiced in knowing she had survived the hospital ordeal and was on the road to recovery. I knew her Alzheimer's disease would never go away, however, as long as she received good physical care and some mental stimulation, she would be OK for a while.

Mammy seemed to be settling well at the Manor on the hill. She was first placed in a room with a terminally ill patient who was fed through a tube. The woman appeared like a mere skeleton on the bed and remained immobile with eyes closed. Mammy made noises and pulled at the curtain on the window above her head, until it eventually had to be removed.

She was thick despite not eating much in the past few weeks, and her arms were quite strong. She looked around the new room with great interest and smiled and sent kisses every time an attendant entered the room.

'Gloria, how are you doing?' the nurse would ask.

'I'm fine,' she would say.

'What's your name? And where are you from?'

'Gloria James from Diamond Vale, Diego Martin,' she would answer.

In 2015, Mammy was still cognisant of her name and the home she owned for over 40 years. She also recognised her car very well after all those years of driving. This brought some relief since she had changed homes and been through some hospital trauma. We always said she was strong as an ox and very stubborn, so this is what took her through the ordeal.

I took pleasure in these simple interactions, as if analyzing a small child. I would give her a newspaper and film her reading the words, not sure if she made any sense of the words she was reading.

With a bit of mischief one morning, she told me that the nurse had hit her.

I asked, 'Did she really do that Mammy?' The nurse looked at her in disbelief.

'Nope,' said Mammy, and sent a kiss to the nurse.

In fact, my mother was the one who had fought the nurse while she tried to seat her in the wheelchair that morning. She was back to her feisty ways but was not mobile anymore. Most days she spent in a wheelchair as she looked at the beautiful, lush vegetation of the mountains. The air was fresh and the dog, Captain, passed every once in a while to say hello.

Characters at the Manor

Colette had already described some of the patients to me. I observed the residents at the Manor with great interest and excitement. The home was relatively new and filled with enthusiastic staff, patients and family members. People brought their loved ones from far and wide to this new and 'revolutionary' home that promised activities and rehabilitation for the elders. It was the dream of the average middle-aged person with no time to take care of their elderly parents. After combing the homes in Trinidad and Tobago for places that provided more than a meal and babysitting with blank stares at a television, we felt as if we'd finally hit the jackpot.

Burt, the owner of the Manor was an enthusiastic registered nurse who studied geriatric nursing in the United Kingdom. Burt was tall, dark and skinny with short curly hair. He wore glasses and a thoughtful smile. Burt was enthusiastic about his role as a caregiver and very good at selling his ideas to nervous, middle-aged 'children', who wanted the best for their parents. The Manor promised weekly music sessions with a visiting guitarist and daily chats and story time with Burt. As with all new enterprises, we hoped they could keep up the standard.

Some of the characters at the Manor included a tall dark man with straight salt and pepper hair, who seemed to have all his senses. He dressed smartly each day and assisted Burt with errands, wearing his dark sunglasses. Saffee, an elderly woman, with a round face, medium length straight grey hair around her face, and wide searching eyes, spoke loudly about how many houses she owned and how she used to sing for a living. She threatened many times to run away to her home in Cocorite and created reasons to 'escape' every day. Her accomplice was a tall and skinny woman with light brown skin, short straight brown hair and early signs of dementia. It was amusing to listen as they plotted their escape home, wherever 'home' was in their minds.

Addee was one of the quiet ones in her 80s. She had suffered a massive stroke and couldn't walk or use her hands. She was thin with olive coloured skin, grey and black short curly hair and large brown eyes. She could speak quite softly to let the nurses know what she wanted. Then there was David a tall dark man with very little woolly hair on his head. He wasn't as old as the others, but somehow ended up at the Manor after a brain operation which affected his ability to think clearly. He had to be observed periodically because he too would walk away very quietly and without warning. A tall, slim man with light brown skin and bulging varicose veins on his legs, came to the Manor wearing a chain with a large crucifix. His claim to fame was that he was a priest. The others called him 'Father' and he prayed with them periodically. His reality may have been different, however, since he swore frequently and had a few choice words for the ladies. Even though he was in his 60s, his former lifestyle gave him the appearance of an 80 year old man. Father craved attention all the time, so he was given tasks to help in the kitchen and around the big house.

Another character was Tyrone, stocky man with light coloured skin, medium length straight black hair and a nose ring worn at the end of his long nostrils. He sat and watched television in his room all day long. He shared a room with an elderly Chinese man who had been paralysed following a stroke.

The big pit bull dog called Captain was tall and a dark brown colour with a broad head. He walked around the house saying hello to all the residents and searching under the table for morsels during lunchtime. Burt said Captain was harmless and friendly. I wasn't convinced. He looked really big to me so I kept a distance and hoped he would be safe and friendly with all the residents, especially my mother.

A tall muscular physiotherapist, Philbert came to do rehabilitation with some of the residents for an extra fee. Philbert looked like a body builder or someone who had consumed a great deal of protein powder and/or steroids. He did a modest trade with the residents and posted every small progress on Facebook so we could observe from afar.

My mother hadn't walked in a year and Philbert promised he could make her walk again with the right exercises. Philbert showed one lady who partially recovered the use of her legs after a stroke and was able to step forward. It was encouraging to watch.

Mammy, who by this time didn't seem to recognise me or other family members, certainly recognised Philbert and we hired him to do exercises with her. He worked with several elderly patients on site so they could exercise and regain some mobility. The nurse told me that Mammy really liked him because he was good looking. The first time he came to do exercises with Mammy, she smiled and winked at him.

When he came into a room, her eyes would light up and she would smile so happily. The same mother, who did not follow the nurses' instructions, would kick out her foot when Philbert asked her to do the exercises. Even in her state of dementia, she knew a good looking man when she saw one, and blushed uncontrollably. She even spoke to Philbert when he asked her to do the exercises. The most miraculous story for us happened when the other patient in Mammy's room died of complications. My mother hadn't been able to utter full sentences to us, and we assumed she wouldn't speak anything that made sense to us again. However, she observed everything that happened around her and listened carefully. Philbert reported that the day after the sick woman's death, he was doing exercises with Mammy and she told him, 'The woman's dead. The woman's dead.'

He was shocked and sent me a message right away. Nobody would have explained anything to my mother when they removed the woman's body from the room. They assumed Mammy was incapable of understanding. This incident demonstrated to me the importance of not ignoring the elderly or speaking badly about them in their presence. One never knew what they could understand or retain. Any statement that could cause pain or unnecessary worry should be avoided.

I pondered the fact that many in our society treated elderly with scorn and spoke badly about them in their presence and wondered how I would cope if my turn came to be in a geriatric hospital or a seniors' home.

## Staff

The location of the Manor was a challenge for staff. The house was so far up the mountain in Maracas Valley St. Joseph that it took three different taxi routes to access. Difficult and expensive access as well as demanding work, made jobs at the Manor unattractive. Staff seemed to stay as long as they could, until another opportunity came.

At first, the main nurse, Sacha held down the fort. She was trained in geriatric care and held a certificate which the resident's families could observe if they wanted in a folder near the front door. The staff also alternated on the night shifts, since 24 hour supervision of residents was required. Nicole, Kizzy, and Tracey, were some of the nurses on duty when I visited. I tried to learn the names so when I called I could speak to the helpers on a first name basis and ask them about my mother's condition. The staff had regular meetings with Burt as he attempted to keep standards high at the home. Luckily, the home had an open door policy and relatives were allowed to visit at any time. They had nothing to hide. This was a refreshing change compared to the last facility

I called regularly from Toronto to get updates from the Manor and the nurse would send WhatsApp videos or Facebook photos and videos to show me how my mother had bounced back from her hospital ordeal. Guilt may have been my motivation, but I constantly looked for cheap flights to return to Trinidad for visits. Even if it was for three days at a time, I would go.

## Routines at the Manor

Residents were served a hot breakfast first thing in the morning. Then everyone was required to take the daily shower, whether they wanted to or not. Those who were able to help themselves were sent to the shower and asked to dress in clean clothes before returning to the sitting room. Those who were immobile were taken out to a backyard in a wheelchair and bathed behind curtains. They were living in a hot country and Burt insisted that everyone got a daily bath. This was a refreshing concept compared to other facilities which would wipe immobile patients daily without giving them that sensation of a shower and shampooing of their hair.

Residents were powdered, dressed and wheeled out to the sitting room to socialize with each other and wait until lunch was served. On some days, a young woman came with a guitar to play songs and get residents to sing and dance. Some were given percussion instruments to play along. A post on Facebook of residents dancing and singing 'Brown Girl in the Ring', really gave me hope that my mother was in the right place and she would live out the rest of her days in a happy environment. Even though my mother could be seen sitting on the sidelines with her head down most of the time, she would occasionally look up, smile at the other residents, and then hang her head back down. I believe she was enjoying the music. Burt was surprised that even though she was a former music teacher, she didn't liven up and participate in the music sessions. Perhaps the disease had ravaged her brain so much; she may not have even remembered her love for music. We would never know.

Burt encouraged a daily story time and rap session with the residents when they could talk about old times or topics that interested them. No one was left out. Even those with advanced cases of dementia or others confined to a wheelchair were brought into the circle to observe and participate. It was different to other homes where the immobile were left in their rooms, as if being punished for not being able to walk. The vocal ones dominated. Others like my mother were still included in the circle, but sat quietly listening. This didn't mean they were not listening to everything.

If nothing else, my mother ate very well. In fact she was always hungry and her brain did not register the fact that she was full. Residents were provided with a well balanced meal at lunchtime: meat or fish with vegetables, a starch and salad. A cook would prepare a balanced meal for lunch every morning and serve all the residents at place settings at the dining table. It was heart warming to see the residents sit and eat together. Those who couldn't sit at the table were fed spoonful by spoonful by one of the patient helpers. Nobody went hungry, which is so important for regaining strength or keeping healthy.

My mother ate every last rice grain on her plate and if the helpers were not looking, she would reach for the plate of any resident near to her, to try to eat his food too. Her hunger knew no bounds.


The Barrel

My mother was in the Manor permanently and Colette had left Trinidad. We couldn't allow the family home to remain idle when it was possible to have another family occupy it. Brent took on the task of massive renovations to make the place rent ready, getting contractors and buying materials. Many household items still remained from Colette's furniture to other family belongings. Decisions had to be made on what could be sold, given away or simply discarded. Colette decided to have several yard sales and advertise to neighbours and the public at large since it would be difficult to re-ship her household goods that she'd previously shipped to Trinidad.

I appointed myself the family historian and felt it my duty to rescue memorabilia which we could never replace. I made a special trip to the house one day when the workmen didn't occupy all the rooms and combed the place for items of sentimental value.

I removed all the family photos and albums, music scores, and wall hangings. Workmen would probably trample over these or they'd end up in the yard with rubble. My parents had collected LPs and 45 vinyl records over the years and I had a few of my own too. Some were warped with time or showed signs of water damage. However, I selected the best in the lot to bring back to Toronto with me. I would have to get a turntable to play them. My parents received countless fine China tea sets as wedding gifts in 1962. Most were destroyed over the years but one partially complete set was saved in the cabinet to be used only on special occasions like Christmas and Easter. I had to rescue my mother's prized fine China set with gold leaf around the rims of the plates and tea cups with tiny painted flowers. A stoneware dinner set with serving dishes, and a set of Pyrex dishes from the 1960s were also salvaged. These were not going to the dump if I had my way.

I informed Brent with great excitement that North Americans enjoyed collecting memorabilia from the 1950s and 60s, including kitchen ware. He just shrugged.

In her hoarding days, Mammy had hidden jewellery by wrapping it in pieces of tissue, then in old socks, and then in pillow cases stuck in cupboards and drawers. It wasn't a good idea to randomly discard items without first shaking them to see if any treasures were in there. Even though we'd removed many valuables like gold bracelets, earrings etc. in the year before, it was still worth checking. I found some beautiful curtains, table cloths and bath mats which I planned to take back with me. My parent's college certificates and diplomas were salvaged. These were excellent examples of family legacy.

After hauling these treasures to the guestroom at Brent's house, I had to find a way to bring everything to my small apartment in Toronto. Colette suggested using a barrel to haul everything by air freight. This was the way many Caribbean people shipped household goods to and from North America. It was the reason why Mammy kept her prized storage barrel for over a decade on one side of the dining room. After working through the myriad of steps on how to get a barrel and ship goods to Toronto, I was able to proceed. The air freight company at the Piarco Airport didn't sell barrels but there was a place on Wrightson Road, in town, where I could get one.

I showed up early one morning and joined the queue for a barrel, borrowing Brent's large pick up truck for the day. People in the queues in Trinidad always stared and seemed nosey, but that day it paid off. I got advice from one person in the line to buy a used barrel instead of a new one. I also learned which window to approach for the purchase. After an elaborate dance, my used barrel was rolled out and I got assistance to load it onto the bed of the pick up truck. Equipped with the barrel I went back home and gingerly wrapped all the Chinaware and stoneware so they wouldn't break in transit. The 44' tall barrel filled up faster than I thought and I wasn't able to fit music scores and some other material. I was leaving the country in two days and not knowing who could collect them at the last minute, unfortunately those items had to go to waste.

I made an appointment with the freight company the next morning and showed up earlier than the staff. When the right person arrived, he said I had to unpack the barrel. They were supposed to look at all the contents to be sure no illegal contraband was being shipped and then sign off on customs documents. My hard work of carefully packing fragile dishes and LPs, and squeezing as much as possible into the 44 inch barrel had been in vain. It was tedious to have to remove everything and then be observed repacking, but it had to be done and a list of goods prepared. Finally a mountain of paperwork was filled and signed and the barrel weighed.

I paid a few thousand dollars to air freight memories to Toronto and clear the goods through Customs. Some would have said I was crazy. However, I felt it was one way of keeping the memories of my parents and family alive. I wanted to hand over these memories to the next generation one day.

In December 2015, Tiffany and I returned to Trinidad to celebrate my mother's 83rd birthday. Tiffany was 19 going on 20. She hadn't seen her grandmother in two years. By that time, Mammy had lost a significant amount of weight, but still had a hearty appetite. When Tiffany first saw Mammy, she held on to me and sobbed uncontrollably.

'Why is she like that? What happened to Granny? Why is she like that? She's so skinny!'

When Tiffany calmed down, I asked her to hug her grandmother and tell her stories and read for her. Granny would have wanted her to be happy.  At least she was still alive. Mammy was a great fighter and survivor.

I invited her friends who were still in touch to come up to the Manor for the birthday celebration, and we bought food to share with all the visitors and the residents. The living room was decorated with banners and balloons and the table was dressed with a happy birthday table cloth. We collected Chinese food from a caterer and a cake was decorated with Mammy's name. When we sang the happy birthday song for Mammy, she looked up, smiled at us, and then hung her head down again. I fed her lunch which she ate heartily and we sat talking about old times until it was time to leave. All the nurses helped with this first birthday party and the residents enjoyed the festivities.

Everything seemed fine for the first six months at the Manor, but then things began to unravel. The head nurse left the job amidst a scandal I could not understand and the helpers continued to run the operations. One by one, I received news that some people removed their parents from the Manor. Even Philbert stopped working with clients at the Manor and attempted to open his own senior's home in an apartment. The whole situation was odd and I was never able to get the whole story from anyone, just gossip and hearsay. The whole fabric of the Manor seemed to have collapsed, even the dog, Captain looked sick when I went back to Trinidad for a visit. Staff members left and new ones were hired, but some faithful ladies remained on staff.

During a short visit to Trinidad, I assessed the facility's practices by visiting at different times, morning and evening, and still felt satisfied my mother would be in caring hands.

'Mammy, will you be OK until I see you again?' I asked.

'Yes Darlin,' she said and gave me a hug and a kiss.

Ten Days Old

We planned Mammy's 84th birthday on December 29th 2016. Fewer residents were present to participate, but we had our ceremonial singing for Mammy and her occasional nod in acknowledgement. Mammy had lost more weight, despite eating mountains of food. The muscles in her legs had atrophied and withered until only skin and bone peered through. She became less vocal and less alert. One thing she never lost was her ability to read and do simple computations.

'Gloria, one and one?' I would ask.

Immediately she would answer, 'Two'.

'Two and two?' I asked.

'Four,' she answered promptly.

One resident still at the Manor was Saffee. She sat with her shoulders slouched as she hung her body in a state of constant depression. Skin hung on her arms that were perhaps once full, now sagging with age. She wore a sleeveless, pink and white cotton house dress which flagged her tiny frame.

'Ten days old I say! Ten days old!' she screamed at the top of her lungs.

Saffee frequently muttered and complained to anyone who would listen. She spoke about home, wherever home was, and wanted to run away home.

'Ten days old! You should be ashamed of yourself!'

One afternoon Saffee complained as she sat at the table looking with disgust at her lunch.

The morning had started quietly. Saffee, Mammy, Father and David had been washed, powdered, and dressed. After breakfast, they sat quietly in the spacious open living room with sofas. A large dining table sat on one side and an open kitchen area was off to the other side. Cool mountain breeze blew through the windows as the radio chimed Christmas songs in the background. Father lurked around with his legs of copious varicose veins. When he spoke he would stick out his tongue uncontrollably.

'Eh, eh. Is like ah have no family. Nobody come to see mih. Is ah long time since dey come to see mih,' moaned Saffee.

'Sometimes ah feel like running away and going home. Oh God, mih fingers hurtin' mih. Is de arthritis yuh know.'

Saffee looked mournfully at her crooked fingers and shed a few tears.

'How could you run away? Where would you go?' I asked to hear what her story would be.

'Ah from Western Main Road in Cocorite. Ah have a house over dere,' she said.

'Oh really,' I continued, wanting to learn more about this home. 'So can you walk home from here? Do you know where to go?' I continued, knowing very well that we were on a mountain many miles from Cocorite and it would not be easy for her to find her way there.

'Is my house! Of course I know de way. Ah will run away!' she continued. 'Ah used to be beautiful yuh know. Ah used to dress up pretty and sing for a livin'. Is my money build dis house!'

She shouted to the sky and told anyone who cared to listen, that she was the reason why they had a seniors' home.

'Ah sing at Carnegie and de band played. Ah was a good singer,' she continued.

'Well, sing something for us,' I challenged. 'Let's hear a nice song.'

'Ah Cyah sing again. Ah too ol',' she moaned. 'Come tomorrow and ah will sing then.'

'But you can still sing I'm sure. How old are you anyway?' I asked.

'Ah must be eighty one. Ah Cyah sing again,' she said

hanging her head, again shedding a few tears.

She lacked the confidence to start a song, so I encouraged her to join in when I sang. I had to think of favourites from her time.

'How about *Unforgettable*?' I asked. 'Do you know that song?'

'Oh yes man. Ah like dat one,' she replied.

And so I started, 'Unforgettable…'

Saffee chimed in, 'Dats what you are…'

Her eyes opened widely and she opened her toothless mouth with glee, head tilted up to the ceiling as she crooned the first phrase.

'Unforgettable…' I continued.

'Both near an' fah…' chimed Saffee.

I didn't know the words and went straight to the chorus, 'That's why darling it's incredible …'

Saffee finished the chorus, 'How someone so unforgettable; Tinks dat I am unforgettable too.'

We clapped for each other as she smiled her toothless smile. Mammy looked up just in time to smile at the end of the chorus, look at everyone, close her eyes and then bend her head down again in quiet reflection.

Since Saffee enjoyed this so much we decided to sing another song. By this time, Father chimed in that he wanted to hear a lively song. It was Christmas time, so I asked if they wanted to sing Christmas carols.

'Yeah man,' said Father.

'Let's sing Jingle Bells,' I said and started singing.

Saffee and Father clapped and sang along with a few words here and there. Saffee no longer seemed to feel pain in her arthritic fingers. The crooked fingers met as she clapped quietly and moved her shoulders backwards and forwards with joy. It was fulfilling to see her so happy with her toothless smile.

When the song was done, I could see them quietly asking for more. Their eyes searched mine for another song and the non-verbal communication was set. The morning had been uneventful thus far, and any interaction brought excitement to their day.

'What would you like to hear?' I asked.

'Oh Holy Night,' said Father. And I got started on this well known Christmas song.

They smiled with glee and Mammy looked up and smiled when I hit a high note.

'Yuh could sing man,' said Father. 'Ah didn't know yuh could sing so!'

The requests came in one by one: Silent Night, Away in a Manger, then Morning has Broken.

I asked them if I could take a break since my voice was getting tired. We let the music from the radio fill the air and turned up the volume.
Saffee moved her shoulders backwards and forwards as lively Soca Parang music blared … 'Sereno, Sereno. Sereno Sera!'

'What time it is dey?' asked Father. 'When we gettin' lunch?'

Mammy looked across at the kitchen anytime someone

passed there. She knew instinctively that her meals came from that wide open kitchen. It was close to midday and usually by that time, one of the nurse helpers would be seen cooking lunch for the residents. Singing songs was a good distraction, but people were getting hungry.

'Don' worry,' said the nurse, 'Burt went to buy lunch. He'll be back soon.'

Burt had driven out and was supposed to return by noon with the lunches, but he was late.

'I hungry oui,' complained Father about ten minutes later. I was getting hungry too and wanted to stay long enough to feed Mammy before leaving the seniors' home to get my own lunch.

'Don' worry. Burt is comin' back just now,' said the nurse.

But Father was worried. He had very little to occupy himself with, and lunch was an important part of the day. They all eagerly looked forward to lunch and I know my mother liked her lunch too.

Eventually Burt arrived with some boxes of fried chicken and chips. The meal was from a popular fast food place and he said he wanted to give the residents a treat. The nurse put out plates and shared the meal then called residents to the table for lunch. I told her I would feed Mammy who was sitting quietly in her wheelchair. Father rose and sat at the table and two other residents joined him. Saffee asked the nurse to help her up since she had been sitting for a long time and couldn't rise easily.

She sat in front of her plate of fried chicken and chips and started to grumble. She held the meat to her mouth and attempted to bite in. Then suddenly a slight grumble turned into a big commotion.

'Stale food, I say! Stale food!' Saffee struggled to get up.

'Saffee sit down and have your lunch!' said Burt.

'You should be ashamed of yourself for giving us dat!' shouted Saffee.

'Ah don' have teeth to eat dat stale food. It hard, hard, hard. Ah not eatin' dat!'

The other residents stared at her silently as they bit into their chicken and took up a few pieces of potato. They were all hungry and that was the meal for lunch, so they had to eat it.

'De res' ah dem won't complain, but not me!' shouted Saffee. 'Ah doh like dat! Stale food!'

She wailed inconsolably, 'Wahhhhhh!!!! Is ten days old. Dat food is ten days old. It too hard.'

'Saffee please settle down and eat your lunch,' said the tiny, young nurse who seemed a bit fragile compared to the five residents put in her charge.

Saffee jumped up from the chair at the dining room table with more energy than usual, and returned to the arm chair in the sitting area with a humpf.

'Ah not eatin' dat. Ten days ol'! Dat food is ten days ol'. You should be ashamed for giving us dat to eat! You should be ashamed!' she shouted at Burt.

Burt looked frustrated and ran around the open kitchen area trying to decide what to do next. In the meantime, I took a knife and fork and was busy cutting up the fried chicken into small bite sized pieces so Mammy could eat the lunch. It was not easy to cut up extra crispy chicken. This had to be held to the mouth and bitten. Since Mammy had very few teeth left, it was also difficult for her to chew the fried chicken. I decided to taste the potato to see what it tasted like. I was not fond of chicken and chips, but many people liked it, so once in a while would be OK, I imagined. The chips tasted like old oil and they were cold. Saffee may have had a point. The meal which was probably tasty when collected at the fast food counter, an hour later was STALE FOOD!

'Saffee do you want bread and cheese,' asked the nurse.

'Waaaaah!' She wailed. 'Now ah have no lunch!'

'Saffee do you want bread and cheese? Come back and sit at the table,' instructed the nurse.

'Stale food! Ten days old! Imagine dat is what you tryin' to feed me. I will not eat it! You should be ashamed of yourself,' she continued.

The nurse helped her back to the table as the elderly men eating sat and focused on their meals.

Saffee looked at the plate of bread and cheese and complained. 'Ah doh like dry bread. Now ah have no lunch. Ah have no lunch! Stale food! Ten days old!'

I remembered we had some left over Chinese food from the previous day in the fridge and decided to heat some of this for Mammy to have lunch she could actually chew.

'Should I heat some for Saffee too,' I asked the nurse.

'Yes, that should be fine,' she confirmed. So I took a nice plate and put out some rice, vegetables, and meat, heating it up for the ladies.

Saffee was still quarrelling and fussing at the table. 'Ah cyah eat dis dry bread. It too dry!'

'Saffee, would you like some of my food?' I asked, as I placed the plate in front of her. 'It's really tasty.'

In her rage, she couldn't even see or enjoy the third meal which was placed in front of her. 'Stale food! Stale food they want to give me here today!'

She flung the plate of Chinese food off the table and cried and wailed again. She lifted her shaking frame to go sit in the arm chair.

'Saffee,' I said. 'You wasted my food. Now I have no lunch and you've flung it to the floor. I could have eaten that.'

'Eh? What?' she paused to listen to me. For a split second, she was able to snap out of her rage.

'That was my lunch I gave you. Now I have no lunch,' I said.

The statement was enough to make her feel guilty and she said she was sorry. I continued to feed Mammy rice and vegetables which she seemed to enjoy. It was easy to chew.

Burt asked Saffee to come to her room and she held his arm while hobbling away quietly out of sight. The other residents finished their meals in silence.


The Touch

By 2017, we could sense my mother's swift demise and possible end. Most of the staff we used to know at the Manor had left and a series of new helpers would come and go, not willing to make the journey or not being committed to this type of difficult work. Only two faithful staff members remained from the original crew. I visited in April when airline prices were affordable. It was as good a time as any to sit with my mother, look at pictures, and read stories. Her body was weak and fragile and her ability to focus was almost gone. I couldn't get any response when I called on the phone so it was better to visit with her in person and hold her skinny hands.

Her eyes sometimes searched mine when I called her name and one time she touched me in recognition while I spoke to Tiffany on the cell phone. It was as if she was saying I should speak to her instead of spending time on the phone.

We all felt the end was near but I still hoped she could hold on longer, just a little longer to celebrate her 85th birthday and meet the New Year.

CHAPTER 8

THE FINAL CHAPTER

Two Birthday Parties

Brent was turning fifty, and Colette and I had planned to be in Trinidad for his birthday party the first weekend of December 2017. His wife planned a grand party at their home with the help of an event planner to coordinate decorations, catering, music etc. I left Toronto a few days before his birthday and Colette flew in from Florida. Since it would be really expensive to fly down to Trinidad a second time to celebrate Mammy's 85th birthday on December 29th, I decided to plan a party for her at the seniors' home on the same weekend. I wanted to celebrate what time she had left on earth. In my mind, any birthday was well worth celebrating.

Colette toyed with the idea of returning to Trinidad after Christmas, but I didn't think it was necessary. The theme for Brent's birthday party was Safari. I bought a leopard print dress for the occasion and Colette was prepared with her camouflage top and skirt. That whole weekend, Colette and I wore Safari themed clothes much to everyone's amusement. We asked to help but the event planner said she had everything under control. I visited Mammy that morning and told her about the big birthday party that night for Brent, but I wasn't sure she understood what was going on. Unfortunately she was not physically fit to attend.

When the party guests rolled in, we noticed people were dressed in fine casual clothes. We were the only ones who observed the theme. Conservative Trinidadians would not observe this theme, but seemed more bent on posing and looking good. They monitored each other's behaviour while the music blared. People stood around the elegantly decorated tables sipping and chatting. My attempts at starting a Conga Line were met with massive resistance.

'Have some behaviour. It's not that kind of party,' I was told.

The night went well with servers presenting elegant hors d'oeuvres, a whole pig roasted in a pit and a sumptuous catered dinner.

Even though we went to bed late, I had a great deal of energy the next day to plan Mammy's birthday party.

'Why are you going through the trouble?' asked Colette.

'Because I want to,' I said.

I would feel riddled with guilt if I hadn't done some kind of celebration for my mother and she died before or around the time of her birthday. My motivation may have been guilt from not living in Trinidad to see her regularly. However, I felt it necessary to celebrate her fragile existence and make sure other's joined me at the party. Many of her friends who were still in contact could not come for one reason or the other. I was very upset with them. Didn't they know that Mammy's birthday party was extremely important? With my single focus, I assumed everyone should drop whatever they were doing to accommodate my own program. Of course this was unreasonable.

Mammy's best friend Kim and her daughter were heading to a Christmas luncheon, much to my dismay. Her other friend, Mennen had a Church engagement and couldn't come. I contacted my friends, Leticia who was in the middle of moving house, as well as Elizabeth who was visiting from Toronto and enlisted their help in party preparations.

I alerted the Manor seniors' home director in advance to have the staff clean the living room, especially the fabric furniture which always seemed to have the lingering smell of the last few residents who sat in them. I bought hors d'oeuvres and a birthday cake at a nearby supermarket, and also got juices and drinks to prepare for Mammy's party. I wanted to get her a little gift, but for someone who could barely speak, couldn't walk, and had little or no appetite, what gift could one possible get?

I headed to the Eastern Main Road just an hour before the party time to find a simple birthday gift at one of the variety stores. My idea was to get a doll to hug or a stuffed toy. On entering a party supplies store, the associate took me around to see their selection of stuffed toys. Eventually I picked a brown teddy bear with a red heart that held the words 'I love you' in front.

The store clerk said, 'I hope your daughter likes the teddy bear.'

It was then I told him the teddy was for my mother who was suffering from Alzheimer's disease and needed something to hug. The young man became visibly shocked and hung his head down. He could barely speak to me after that. I was surprised to see the effect these words had on him.

'Don't worry,' I said. 'She's like a big child. She would love the teddy bear. Don't feel sad for her. Thanks for helping me.'

How could he feel so sad for a total stranger? This made me feel like crumbling and crying for my mother too. She had been such a tough woman in her youth and was now reduced to having a childlike mind and body with Alzheimer's disease. I paid the bill swiftly and left. We were celebrating another birthday, and it had to be done with gusto.

I met two friends and we made our way up the mountain one more time to see Mammy. The staff was waiting for us. The nurses and helpers had cut up fruits I had brought the day before. According to my instructions, the living room looked tidy. Flies still could be seen attacking the fruit covered with plastic film, and landing on crumbs on the sofa. It was a lost battle.

We fixed the table with decorations, cake and party food while the residents looked suspiciously over the partition that separated the living room from the TV room. They anticipated the refreshments to follow. Four nurse helpers were present that day; more than usual because the head nurse was away. One of the helpers dressed Mammy and brought her to the living room in a wheel chair.

I waited a while to see who else would show up. Deborah, Mammy's God daughter came, and Colette and Brent arrived later with drinks and ice. That was our little party crowd. The girls wheeled Mammy out to the living room and she held her head down most of the time, appearing quite drowsy. She wore a red and white Batik party dress.

'Gloria. Gloria! Happy Birthday! We're having a party for you,' we said. She would only lift her head when we called her name.

Poor Mammy may have been in pain, but we would never know. She opened her eyes, looked around briefly smiling, and then hung her head back down.

I presented her with the stuffed toy and she looked at it and smiled. Before I knew it, Mammy bit into the face of the teddy bear. Like a baby who puts everything in her mouth, she was actually biting the teddy bear. If we didn't laugh, we would cry.

'No Mammy, no. Don't bite the teddy,' I screamed. 'Just hug it.'

I tried to make her hug the toy, but this was in vain. She may have been hungry or just acting on instinct. Again, we would never know. Colette gave her a bunch of flowers saying, 'Happy Birthday Mammy.'

She held the flowers and must have bitten into them when we were not looking, because we saw petals falling out of her mouth. The gift giving was turning out to be a disaster, but we were not deterred. We sang the Happy Birthday song loudly and with the help of my friends and some of the staff, we cut up the cake, fixing plates of food for all the residents of the home who sat in the TV room. I tried feeding Mammy puffs, sandwiches and cake. She ate her party food heartily while the flies attacked the spoils on the table as well as everyone in the room.

Leticia was disgusted by the flies and spent a great deal of time covering food so they couldn't touch it.

The owner of the Manor must have asked all the staff to be on site for Mammy's party, probably expecting a large crowd. They all sat around looking slightly resentful when they could have been home resting on a Sunday. In the end, only six of us were on hand and not much extra help was needed.

After an hour or so, the party was done and we helped clean the table and clear everything away. One of the attendants wheeled Mammy swiftly to the bedroom. I noticed she was a little rough in wheeling her out and a wheel ran over my mother's foot. Mammy screamed out in pain and it broke my heart. What else could happen when I was not around? What a horrible existence, depending on strangers to bathe you, feed you, move you around, and take care of your every need? I wondered if I would want to live like that. It was certainly a risky existence because one had to depend on the integrity of the staff and possibly their mood in doing a very difficult job.

I helped the nurse to put my mother in her bed, gave her a hug, then loaded up some of the left over supplies and headed back down the hill in the car. I felt just a little satisfied to know that we celebrated another of Mammy's birthdays. Nobody knew if she would be alive to see another one.

The next day I visited Mammy, it was to say goodbye before I headed back to Toronto. This was always difficult, because in her precarious condition, I thought it would be the last time I saw her alive.

I showed her photos from her family book, and pictures in an album. Then I gave her a big hug. She looked at me and smiled, not quite understanding when I said, 'Take care yuh hear? I want to see you again.'

'Ah seeing yuh tomorrow?' asked Mr. Bradford, who always hovered when anyone came to visit a relative.

'Perhaps,' I said.

I didn't want anyone to know I was leaving the next day. Let them imagine I would be back for a visit. There was no harm in showing up unannounced.


Let Her Eat Cake

Mammy's ever faithful friend, Kim had made up her mind to go visit on her birthday, December 29th. Kim and her daughter planned a little party for Mammy. The drive up the hill to the Manor was precarious, so Kim's daughter volunteered to drive up the hill and prepare for the party. They took cake, decorations and flowers and told us they were going at lunchtime. From their reports and photos, it was not a happy sight. Mammy's eyes were permanently closed and Kim described the Mammy was travelling to the other side. The staff dressed Mammy in one of her red house dresses and wheeled her out to the living room to interact with her guests. She was seated on the sofa with her one sick leg permanently bent up and immobile. The other leg was extended and unable to bend. The front of her hair was pulled into a pony tail. She breathed slowly and did not speak, except to grunt in acknowledgement when her name was called.

'Gloria. Gloria. Happy Birthday,' said Kim.

'Hmm,' was her reply.

Not being phased by the situation, Kim and her daughter sang the Happy Birthday song and cut up the homemade black fruit cake they had brought, decorated with the number 85 and red cherries. Kim fed Mammy some cake and she chewed continuously, not once opening her eyes. After about an hour had passed and with little else to do, they said farewell, and Mammy was taken back to her room to lie down.

Brent and his family also decided to go to visit Mammy on her birthday that evening. They piled into one car and set out for the Manor. On their way, Brent got a call from staff saying Mammy was having difficulty breathing and was not eating with her normal gusto. She had been rushed to the emergency ward of Mount Hope Hospital. I got notified in Toronto and went into panic mode. Was this it? Was this the end? Nothing bad was supposed to happen on a birthday. A birthday was supposed to be a happy time. How could this happen? I called my brother continuously for updates, but he couldn't give any. All we knew was that the hospital was doing tests.

My brother went to the emergency ward the following day to see Mammy who was hooked up to an oxygen line and saline solution being fed through an intravenous drip. I remembered the dire conditions at that emergency ward from several years before. Busy hospital staff were too bothered to speak to family members. Lunchroom staff dropped off food only to patients who were able enough to feed themselves. It was a nightmare. I could only imagine how cold and afraid my mother must have been, alone in the emergency ward. Nobody could be expected to stay forever with her in emergency while they waited for 'news', I harassed the nurse from the seniors' home and also my brother for information via WhatsApp, until they were probably tired of me.

The following day, Mammy was discharged from the hospital and the senior's home staff collected her from the hospital. When pressed for information about what was wrong with her, nobody could tell me. The hospital had done blood tests and a CT Scan...

And...

That was the problem with living far away. Nobody seemed motivated to chase the hospital staff for results of the tests, and everybody was super busy. All I could do was call and follow up hoping for some news. Colette said she was thinking of flying down right away. I told her, if the hospital discharged Mammy, she must have been OK. I was not going to fly down to Trinidad unless it was absolutely necessary. I wasn't sure what I would be doing if I flew down to Trinidad anyway. Was I going to be on death watch? I found that idea revolting. Was I supposed to look at my mother until she died? I decided to stay put. Colette started looking at ticket prices. She was a teacher and classes were not scheduled to start back until January 8th after the Christmas break, so she had free time.

## Come On Time

'You have to come on time. Make sure you come on time,' said a good friend who lives in Trinidad.

What was this obsession with arriving to watch a parent die?

She told me hysterically, 'My brother was not able to come on time when our mother died.'

I wasn't sure if I really wanted to arrive 'on time' to watch my mother die. I didn't think I would have the nerve to observe this, especially if it was a painful death. I had watched too many movies in the past.

On January 1st I received a WhatsApp message Burt saying that Mammy was found on the floor and had apparently fallen off the bed at night. She was rushed to the emergency ward at Mount Hope General Hospital again. They were not taking any chances because he felt they did not have the necessary equipment and means to take care of her. I found it difficult to understand. How could she fall off the bed when she was barely able to move?

That was the 'deal breaker' for Colette. She booked her ticket for a week to travel down to Trinidad hoping to return before her job started back. I was looking at airline tickets, but again didn't want to rush back home.

'My mother is dying,' wailed Colette. 'I bought her a dress.'

'What?'I asked. 'Why did you buy her a dress? She has so many dresses at the home already.

'Are you kidding?' said Colette. 'She has to look good in the coffin. She doesn't have anything nice in the cupboard at the Manor. It's peach with a shimmer and has a short sleeved jacket. '

That statement made me recoil in horror.

Not only was she going to visit my mother, but she was already planning the funeral in her head and how she would dress Mammy as if this was some sort of party.

I could barely speak …

'You're in denial. You know she's going to die and you won't admit it! Well you can stay right there and dream on. I have a gut feeling this is it I know these things!' she went on and on.

Colette called me within an hour saying she'd bought her ticket and was ready to go down.

'You're in denial. She's going to die. She's going to die. You have to be prepared,' she wailed.

In my mind, my mother was not dead until pronounced dead and I still had hope that somehow she would recover from this trip to the hospital, just like all the other episodes.

The bad news about having a weak immune system and resting in the emergency ward for days was the risk of picking up infections from all the other patients.

I decided to wait a week and just call Brent, Burt, Colette, and everybody for news, even if it drove me crazy.

I booked my ticket for Monday 8th January 2018 to go to Trinidad. I was to arrive late on Monday night.

Hospital Drama – Day 1

The flight was uneventful and I camped in the guest room at my brother's house as usual. That night I could hardly sleep in anticipation of going early to the hospital to speak with a doctor. Getting to see a doctor was usually a tricky dance at hospitals in Trinidad. Nurses never gave information, so I knew I had a put on a suit of armour with plenty of patience in order to find out about my mother's condition. My brother said he had been lucky to speak to a doctor the previous day. We set out around 8 am to catch the doctors when they did their early morning rounds.

My mother was given a bed in Ward 9 which was behind the Children's Ward. The hospital grounds looked clean and spacious and as we approached the Ward, we could see patients through the open louvers. There were six beds in the room where my mother rested and Brent pointed out her bed close to the window on one side of the room. I couldn't really see her. She was tiny with a sheet covering her and two bags of drips hung from a pole. A security guard sat at the closed main doors to that wing. We told security our mother was a patient and we were coming to speak to a doctor when they did their rounds. She instructed us to let the people at the nursing station know and then wait in the waiting room at the side. Visiting hours started later at 11 am.

I could not imagine waiting in a waiting room right next to my mother's room and not being able to run in and speak to her. Should I be obedient and sit in the waiting room or should I break the rules and risk being put out? I was not sure what to do. Hospital security could be a nice or as belligerent as they chose to be. I decided to abide by the rules and stay in the waiting room, just looking into my mother's room in hope. Brent had to rush back home since a repair man was coming to the house. I notified the nurse at the station that I was waiting to see my mother's doctor and she said, it was no problem and wrote it in a big hard cover notebook. The nurse's station had about four nurses and nurses' aids dressed in different coloured uniforms, writing copious notes about Lord knows what. I sat watching the dynamics as staff came and went.

The waiting room had about fifteen black chairs and a small washroom off to one side. The place looked clean and smelled clean, which was a great relief. One person mopped the hallway with bleach then reached the waiting room to do her mopping. I stepped into the hallway briefly and peeped through the louvers of my mother's room to see one young woman on the bed near the doorway. My mother's body was motionless on the bed with a bony hip sticking up as she lay on her side. On the other side of the room were three beds. A young girl paced back and forth near the bed at the window. A special needs young woman sat motionless on her bed in the middle staring at the wall. A new patient was brought into the room and was given instructions by two attending young doctors.

What I noticed most was the youth parading as doctors. Or was this because I was middle aged and older than everyone? The doctors seemed fresh out of high school. They distinguished themselves from the nurses, because they did not wear uniforms, and they each sported a stethoscope around the neck like a badge of honour. Doctors came and went and I became anxious. I went back to the nurses' station and enquired if the doctor for Gloria James was coming any time soon. I had been waiting one hour. The new person I spoke to didn't seem aware that I was waiting for a doctor and said she would try to reach him. She started making phone calls. This was really upsetting. They may have changed staff and nobody knew what I what talking about.

A young woman went to my mother's beside, took some vital signs, and wrote notes on a chart. I approached her as she came out the room and said, 'That's my mother. I'm visiting from Canada. What is her condition?'

The woman seemed shocked that I would ask her a question. She gave me a dead pan stare and said I was to wait in the waiting room until the doctor arrived. So there I was, back to square one, waiting in the room for the doctor to come. When the visiting hour of 11 am approached, more people joined me in the waiting room. A woman said she had come to get a death certificate for her nephew who died the night before and she wasn't quite sure what documents were required. I was shocked by the word death certificate and could barely speak to her. Finally at two minutes to 11 am I walked in the room to see my mother.

She looked mournfully fragile with a plastic mask over her nose and mouth and hooked up to the oxygen supply on the wall so she could breath. Mammy lay on one side with the bent leg still bent and her bony hip covered but protruding through the sheet. Both arms were spread akimbo and numerous pieces of cotton and bandages could be seen on her wrists and arms where she had been stuck multiple times, I assumed to find a vein. Two bags of drips hung on poles next to the bed; one for saline solution and another for glucose. A clip board was attached to a little tray and this is where the nurse's aid wrote the vital signs periodically – heart rate, pulse, level of saline and sugar.

'Mammy I came to see you,' I said, and kissed her forehead.

Her eyes were firmly shut and she breathed heavily. I touched her heel, but there was no reaction. Colette arrived in time for visiting hours. She had been staying with a neighbour near our childhood home Colette suggested just holding her hands and we would sit and watch her.

And that's what we did until 1 pm, the end of the morning visiting hours. We went to find something to eat until visiting hours opened up again from 4pm – 6 pm. It was a torturous time of not knowing what to do and just waiting.

My mother's sister Audrey and her husband had recently arrived from Florida and came to visit Mammy that afternoon. They both looked skinnier and more fragile since the last time I saw them. They hobbled across the courtyard as they approached the ward and Aunt Audrey spoke incessantly.

'Who are you again?' she asked.

'I'm Lindy and that's Colette,' I said.

She didn't recognise us and we hadn't spoken to her for a long time because we were not pleased with her erratic behaviour over the past three years. It became apparent at that moment she was showing signs of dementia, possible Alzheimer's disease. It ran in my mother's family and there was no escaping.

'Who are you again?' she asked two or three times again. Even if she didn't know us, she knew her sister, Gloria.

She cried for our Mammy and created a bit of drama. We talked about old times and Audrey said prayers for Mammy while Kenrick went off to buy bottles of cold water and little hotdogs at the visitor's cafeteria nearby. He reminded us repeatedly that we should call our aunt. After seeing her mental state, I felt a bit guilty for not following up with her to see how she was doing over the last few years.

Kenrick explained he had to do everything for her since she was losing her memory and unable to take care of herself. Aunt Audrey loved to dress beautifully all her life, and so even though her mind was deteriorating she wanted to wear her makeup. Kenrick found her that very day putting nail polish on her lips. When he relayed the story, Aunt Audrey chimed in, 'Don't bother with him. Nothing's wrong with that!'

He really had his hands full because she was quite argumentative.

Before we knew it, the security guard rang a bell to alert everyone it was 6 pm and time to leave. We dragged our feet slowly out of the ward and promised to meet again at Mammy's bedside the next day. The doctor never came that day. When I enquired at the nurses' station on a new evening shift, I learned that doctor had passed early that morning around 6:30am and was not coming until the following morning. They could have told me that when I was there at 8:00 am. It was just one of the frustrations of manoeuvring through the medical system.

Hospital Drama – Day 2

On Wednesday morning I went early again to try to speak to a doctor and find out what tests had been done and what my mother's prognosis was like. My mother lay in the same position on one side, breathing with the assistance of the oxygen mask. She was motionless. Colette said she would collect Audrey and Kenrick and bring them to the hospital. We were afraid they'd collapse from walking in the hot sun and pass away faster than Mammy. Colette vowed only to do the morning visit that day since she had been to the hospital several days in a row before we all arrived in Trinidad, I had nothing to do and no place to go but to spend time at my mother's bedside, so I didn't mind. The nurses promised I would see a doctor sometime that day, but they were not sure exactly when. So it was another vigil to get information. Colette, Audrey, Kenrick and I entered Mammy's room just before 11 am and took our seats completely ignoring the sign which read '2 visitors per patient'. We had travelled from far away and couldn't possibly be made to follow that rule. We made a great deal of noise in discourse around Mammy's bed and suddenly she moved her body just a little. I told them, 'You see, you are all making too much noise. Mammy's probably thinking that we should all shut up!'

We had a good laugh which was good to break the sombre atmosphere. I noticed that a young woman dropped off food for each patient at breakfast time on a tray at the bedside. Only those conscious enough to use the spoon and eat availed of this food. This excluded my mother. The girl came at lunchtime and removed the breakfast container and placed another container of liquid lunch at her bedside. I asked her why she was dropping off the container of food and who was going to feed my mother.

She said that was not her job. Her job was just to drop off the food assigned for each patient. It was up to the nurses to feed them. I enquired at the nurses' station and they feigned ignorance saying somebody was supposed to feed my mother. It was the same thing I noticed the day before, unopened Styrofoam cups with a little liquid in them. How could a patient hope to recover without nutrients? I noticed the special needs young woman opposite, and she also had several unopened food containers at her bedside. Nobody had bothered to feed her and she was young. I knew very well that the elderly would be ushered to their demise without conscience in many situations, but was there no mercy for a young person? Why would people even go into the nursing profession if they didn't care about others?

At lunchtime, the thoughtful security guard told me about a cafeteria upstairs I could visit because they had better food than the one downstairs. I left the group briefly to eat something since I'd been waiting since early morning to get to speak to a doctor. When I entered the cafeteria on the second floor of the adjacent building, I noticed only nurses in uniforms and young doctors with their stethoscopes around their necks were in the room. Several fast food and full meal options were available and there was even a TV screen showing foreign programs on one side of the room. This was such an upgrade to the poorly stocked, tiny café available to the public on the ground floor. It was the staff canteen.

I bought a full meal and sat down to eat being famished from arriving on site early. Many of the nurses stared at me, probably wondering if I was a new staff member. They stared and stared but couldn't figure out my story. I hustled through my meal and while eating got a call that the doctor was at Mammy's bedside and I was to come back right away. Of course the minute I disappeared was when he arrived.

I rushed back downstairs with my list of questions.

The doctor was another young one like the myriad of youngsters I'd seen with stethoscopes. He was accompanied by another young doctor and told me about the tests that were done. He advised that my mother had suffered multiple strokes and would probably never recover enough to talk and function normally. He also suggested that the hospital was not the place for long term care and we should consider palliative care.

Oh the dreaded words, 'Palliative Care'. That meant waiting to die.

I had to come to terms with the fact that my mother was dying, but she moved that day. When Brent came to the hospital and scratched her heel, she twitched her leg. Wasn't that something? Wasn't this a sign that she could recover? Why were people so eager to give up on the elderly? Mammy had been through a lot, in and out of hospital many times. I was convinced that if we could afford the best health care, she would bounce back. However, nobody else had that notion. She had a wretched existence unable to walk for two years, with one foot permanently bent from lack of use.

Her body was that of a skeleton and had been that way for two years. It was really a terrible way to live. The doctor suggested a palliative care facility at Caura Village. We listened carefully to the options. He said the doctor in charge would come to visit the hospital on Friday and he could refer Mammy to their facility. If the facility had a bed available, they could take my mother right away. He explained that we would have to agree to no feeding and no resuscitation.

All family members seemed to agree with this. I hesitated… This meant letting my mother die naturally without the assistance oxygen and without any nutrition to keep her alive.

Would this be painful for her? How could I agree to something like that? It would hasten her death and I would feel responsible. The guilt would destroy me.

The doctors left and we had a lot to ponder.

At the same time, staff from the Manor seniors' home arrived to see Mammy; Burt and two of his nurses. They hugged her and hugged all the family. Then one nurse said I smell something. They checked, and Mammy had not been cleaned and changed. I alerted the chatty nurse's aid who had been walking around the ward all morning.

'How come you didn't change my mother this morning?' I accused her. 'And look at this plastic mask for the oxygen. The mask is digging into her eye socket. Just because a patient can't speak doesn't mean you people should treat them badly!'

I was hysterical because I had only then noticed the top part of the mask digging into my mother's left eye. How many times had someone taken her vital signs like a robot and not bothered to even look at her to see if she was comfortable? I doubted that I would ever want to be a helpless patient in a hospital. The thought was frightening.

The nurse's aid apologized and said she was doing the rounds and was getting to my mother soon. I'm not sure how genuine this was. Luckily the staff from the Manor cleaned and dressed Mammy while the nurse's aid looked bothered and confused. They had brought extra clothing for her to wear since everything she had in the hospital was now dirty. They were accustomed to taking care of Mammy so we left the room and let them do their job. The nurse's aid who probably felt slighted came to whisper to me that Mammy had bed sores and she came to the hospital just like that. It was the fault of the people at the senior's home. Well, I noticed that the hospital staff never turned my mother in the two days I was there, so her gossip didn't matter. That would surely have caused serious bed sores!

We thanked the staff from the Manor for taking good care of Mammy for the past three years and extending her life as best as they could with loving care. We all gave Mammy a farewell hug and parted ways.

A Gentle Resting Place

I can't even remember my last words to my mother when I left her that afternoon with the big group.

I called my friend Joyanne to tell her what transpired and she offered to take me to the Palliative Care facility in Caura. She arrived in a short time and off we went, with no appointment, just a mission to see the place and learn about their program.

The grounds of the Palliative Care facility were in the foothills north east of the hospital. It was a spacious and airy location with many mature trees in the yard. The old buildings were British colonial style and brightly painted. Security made no fuss. We said we were visiting the Palliative Care facility and they just said go ahead. That was too easy. When we walked into the main entrance, we said we were visiting the facility and would like to speak to a doctor. The attendant called the doctor who was responsible for the facility. It was a young Asian woman and luckily, she made time to speak with us. I told her about my mother's condition.

She explained that Palliative Care was supposed to be short term, providing pain killers and comfort until a patient died. I saw a few people on beds in the facility and it hit me that they were all waiting to die. How could this really nice doctor work in a Palliative Care facility?  I guess it was a necessary evil and someone had to do it. She reminded me that their policy was *No Feeding and No Resuscitation*. I would have to sign an agreement with their policy and she cautioned many family members were not comfortable with this. She also said it was possible to keep a corpse alive for months on oxygen and drips, but if this was what I wanted, then they would not do it.

The facility was clean and comfortable. I was satisfied that if my mother were admitted, it would have been a comfortable resting place until the end.

## CHAPTER 9

## FUNERAL PLANS

The Call

I had a restless sleep that night, thinking of everything that transpired during the day. Early next morning, Thursday 11th January, 2018, Brent woke me up saying he got a call from the hospital and we were to dress and go right away. I threw on some clothes, fixed my hair and away we went.

'What did they say? What did they say?' I asked frantically.

'Nothing; just to come right away,' he said.

I called Colette and she said she would try to get there soon, but would meet traffic on the way from Diego Martin to Mt. Hope.

We got to the hospital, parked and rushed to the ward. I saw a curtain drawn around Mammy's bed. Just then a nurse's aid popped out carrying a basin in her hands. What was going on? What did this all mean? We went to the nurse's station and they said we should wait in the waiting room until the doctor arrived. It was the usual annoying drill, to sit around with no information. Of course she didn't know when the doctor would come, just that we had to wait.

Brent and I speculated that Mammy may have died. After all, the curtain was drawn and no other patient had curtains drawn.

What was going on?

When Colette came she did not want us to sit waiting for the ever passing doctor. She suggested going en masse to the nurse's station to find out what was happening.

Colette got loud, 'Excuse me. Can you tell us what's happening with patient, Gloria James?'

The nurse said, 'Ma'am can you all please sit in the waiting room? The doctor is on his way.'

'Listen if our mother is dead, just tell us! What is this madness? Just tell us so we will know. The curtain is drawn, so we can guess anyway!'

With the ranting and shouting, the nurse admitted that our mother had died in the wee hours of the morning. She never gave a specific time. She said when the doctor came, he would provide more information.

It was the inevitable. We didn't have to wait for a bed to become available in the Palliative Care facility in Caura. Mammy didn't have to endure another day on the ventilator and not being fed or changed. She didn't have to live with a permanently bent leg and the inability to walk, while bedsores destroyed her flesh. There was no more pain from arthritis in her joints. She no longer had to endure the horrible catheter to remove urine or the needles destroying her wrists and arms to deliver fluid to her skeletal body. I imagined it must have been a relief to be out of that shell of a body.

Even though it was painful to know our mother had died, in some ways, it was comforting to know she would no longer suffer.

No more pain.

The doctor came swiftly and described that she had died in the night. He prepared the documents we would take to register Mammy's death at the registrar on site at the Mount Hope Complex. The document said Mammy died of aspiration pneumonia, a cardio vascular accident, diabetes mellitus, and atrial fibrillation.

We were finally allowed to go in and say a final farewell to Mammy.

I felt afraid to enter through the drawn curtain, not knowing exactly what I would see. I was shaking like a leaf.

There she lay lifeless and covered up to her neck. She looked really tiny on that twin sized bed. A woman who used to be big and strong was reduced to a mere shadow of her self. We all cried and I hugged Colette, and then I hugged Brent. Our poor Mammy was finally gone and nothing could bring her back. Brent said a prayer for her from his Bible. I kissed her forehead and after a short time, we all left.

I felt a strange sense of emptiness that still lingers, even today. No longer was I going to be able to call her at the Manor to get a little conversation of schwim and schwam, or a kind 'Yes Dahlin'. No longer would I be able to call the seniors' home to find out how she was doing. I wouldn't have to frantically look for airline deals to Trinidad, so I could run away for a quick visit. My life was going to change drastically.

Planning Mammy's Funeral

Hospital staff was going to move Mammy's body to the morgue and we were responsible for making arrangements with a funeral home to collect her body.

Colette, Brent and I needed to immediately change from grieving mode to planning mode. We couldn't allow ourselves to wallow in grief that day. Colette had taken an extra week off work and I had to call and reschedule a job the following week. We both had to cancel flights and rebook new flights, leaving days later.

A list of funeral preparation steps was hastily prepared and we divided the responsibilities. We also wanted to plan a memorable funeral and send off for our mother. With very little time on our hands, we had to do this quickly. It was already Thursday 11th January and we wondered how soon we could get a priest to officiate at the funeral at St. Michael's and All Angels.

Colette dropped me off at the registry of births and deaths on the Medical Campus, to register Mammy's death. Brent went home to get documents for the funeral home and cemetery. Colette tried to get information on the church and made an appointment at their office that day. She had to secure the church and priest, propose a program, and book the parish hall for the reception.

It was still early morning at the Registry of births and deaths. When I joined the queue, it was not long. Happily I had the required documents from the hospital and identification in the form of my passport which I carried that morning. I signed documents to register Mammy's death and the whole experience seemed surreal. I felt like a huge weight was on my shoulders as her first born child. While I was inside, Colette managed to contact the church office and secured a date of Monday 15th January, when the priest was available to preside over the funeral. That was great news. If we could get the funeral home to make all the arrangements and announce the funeral for us, that would give us a chance to return to work and other obligations.

We had little time to mourn, and no time to grieve. I believe we had mourned the loss of our mother during the prior three years when she was in the late stages of Alzheimer's disease. The mother we used to know had slipped away slowly, day by day, leaving a shell.

We all went downtown to apply for the death certificate at the Civil Registry, the government office responsible for issuing the death certificate, which was on South Quay in Port-of-Spain. I went into the large, crowded hall and received a number, joining one queue, and then the next. This office worked efficiently and I was impressed at their precision in processing applications for certificates of marriages, births and deaths. People paid and received a beautifully printed certificate in minutes. The sign at the cash register read 'Cash Only. Provide Exact Change'. I thought to myself that they couldn't be serious with that rule. So many people were coming in with cash, so they must have change when I got to the front.

Well, I was wrong. The cashier sent me away, 'Go and get cash and come back. Next!'

I was shocked at her stern nature and the way she moved on to the next person in line with no emotion or concern. The few customers I asked in the line for change didn't have any to give. One man suggested I go to the food vendors opposite the building, and buy a little something to get change. That was what I had to do, and returned to order two copies of Mammy's death certificate. The certificates were printed immediately using information already entered in the database at the regional Registry at Mount Hope. I was impressed at the efficiency of the whole process, when some other government services did not run so well.

With death certificate in hand, we then went to the funeral home to make arrangements. Brent had become quite skilled in planning funerals, having arranged my aunt's and my father's funerals single-handedly while we lived abroad. We found parking in the tiny yard at the funeral home and spoke with the amicable staff. They provided very good customer service. Never had I expected people in the business of death to be so friendly. They helped us choose a casket, plan the cover for the program, create wording for a death announcement, and set up announcements in local newspapers, starting on Friday 12th January. The funeral home detailed what we needed to bring the following day. We chose a simple cherry coloured casket with brass handles. I didn't like the idea of a large gaudy box. None of us thought this was necessary.

The funeral home wanted to know exactly where to collect Mammy's body and Colette let them know she had already prepared Mammy's burial dress. The attendant said they liked to dress up the deceased as if they were going to a wedding. We had to provide stockings, underwear, jewellery; and everything except shoes. I found this concept extremely bizarre. Why did we dress up the dead in the finest clothes? I wondered where this tradition originated. Certainly ancient cultures were known to do this with royalty. We made a down payment and promised to return the next day with the balance and outstanding material.

Brent and I went to visit the Lapeyrouse Cemetery to make our reservation for a Monday burial and Colette headed to Diego Martin to visit the church.

Lapeyrouse Cemetery was like a little town in the middle of the district of Woodbrook. The Cemetery streets were named with well marked graves and tombstones, as well as simple unmarked graves where crumbling flowers could be seen. The manager had a detailed map of Lapeyrouse Cemetery, one of the oldest in Trinidad and Tobago, and steeped with history. Generations of past inhabitants of Port-of-Spain were buried there and plots were left as a legacy in families. Brent remembered vaguely where my aunt was buried many years before, and Mammy was going to be buried in the same plot. He had all the documents for the location on hand and the manager went into her files to search for the plot. She asked if we needed a six foot or a nine foot grave. We didn't know the significance of this, but learned that with a six foot grave, nobody could be buried in that spot for at least nine years to allow the newly buried corpse time to fully decompose. She suggested we aim for a morning funeral and arrive at the Cemetery on Monday before the grave diggers went for lunch break or finished work for the day. Any delay would mean paying overtime fees.

Discussing the plot where Mammy's body would be laid to rest was another surreal experience for me. I felt numb and with no emotion. It felt like a business transaction and I somehow wondered if we were being callous and just talking business. Brent and I went with the lead grave digger to look for the plot but couldn't find it. I thought that my grandmother's name would be on the tombstone but we didn't see anything. Even though we provided a plot number, the grave digger said he would have to look at a map more closely for the exact spot on Monday morning to know where to dig. Burial plots ran in different directions, not just one direction. According to him, we could have been standing on the plot and not know it, if there was no head stone. At least I knew the approximate location of the site in reference to a school building on Tragarete Road outside the cemetery walls. I made a mental note to use this school as a reference when visiting Mammy's gravesite in the future years.

We went back up to Mount Hope Hospital to identify Mammy's body at the morgue and get the exact location to inform the funeral home for collection. I let Brent go in with the doctor's paperwork to identify the body. I became squeamish and horribly afraid of the fact that naked bodies were placed like slabs of meat in freezers awaiting burial or cremation. Worse again, the thought of looking at Mammy's body was terrifying. The indignity of the whole process made me sick. Poor Brent had been through this process before, seeing my aunt's dead body and also my father's dead body. I couldn't imagine his terror, but just didn't want the responsibility. When he came out, he said the attendant would not let him look at Mammy's feet only, even though he could recognise Mammy's feet. He was forced to look at the whole body, including her head. Poor Brentos... I felt so sorry for him, while I shook in fear, standing outside the door, hiding my face in my hands. Alas, it was all over.

Brent immediately called the funeral home with the exact location and number for Mammy's body in the morgue, so they could go collect it. The funeral home charged a rental fee based on the number of days they housed a body and the list of fees was quite long.

When we returned to Brent's home, he hastily planned a reception that night for friends to visit. I called a few people whom I remembered in the spur of the moment, and forgot many others.

My main focus had switched to planning the order and content of the service. I had to send an email to the funeral home on the next day so they could print programs for us. I also had to change my flight and book a ticket for Tiffany to travel to Trinidad for her Granny's funeral. She felt her university class on the Tuesday night was a priority and she didn't want to miss it. In addition, I managed to reschedule a two day consulting job towards the end of the week. So much planning was needed and my poor head was buzzing. That evening, I was glued to my laptop and Brent kept reminding me to speak to guests when they arrived for the Wake. I was in an antisocial state and really didn't want to speak to anybody. What could I possibly tell them? I just wanted quiet time that evening to get my life and the funeral plans in order, but people kept arriving at the house.

I came out to the living room reluctantly with my laptop and sat there planning, while Colette entertained some friends and Brent spoke with his friends. Now and then, I looked up as Mammy's good friend Kim recalled funny escapades when she and Mammy worked together as high school teachers. In my head, I was planning a grand musical performance of Fauré's Requiem for Mammy's funeral. The Requiem by Gabriel Fauré is a beautiful Requiem sung in four parts: soprano, alto, tenor, and bass. Even though the Requiem is about 35 minutes long and appears deceptively simple, it wasn't easy to sing. I realised I would have to get some experienced singers to perform this. The average church choir wouldn't usually take on such a demanding piece of music.

I asked for singers from a choir I used to sing with while living in Trinidad. However, the director said they had stopped doing funerals, since choir members couldn't get time away from work. Joyanne put me in contact with the music director of a University choir and I sent him a message immediately. Fortunately his choir had performed the Fauré the year before, and so the students knew the music. Since students were still on vacation, he promised to send email messages to get them out on a busy Monday morning to perform. The email was sent and I crossed my fingers and hoped for the best.

The church asked Colette if we wanted a traditional mass or not. Colette opted for the traditional mass with communion and I used the template they provided to intersperse movements from the Fauré and make things fit as best as I could. An opportunity was created for one grandchild from each family to do a reading and each sibling to do a tribute or eulogy. Many family photos of Mammy in her younger years and photos with children and grandchildren were assembled so the funeral home staff could create a collage in the middle pages of the program. For the front page, I chose a beautiful black and white portrait of Mammy, probably taken in the 1960s. I had spotted this photo in an old family album rescued from the house when everything was being removed.

We were supposed to send back the program to the priest

for approval, but this never happened. I tried calling a few people to tell them about the Monday funeral, but that was an onerous task and I missed many people. We hoped they would see the announcement in the newspapers and just show up. I also put a funeral announcement on my Facebook page with an appeal for good singers.

On Friday, we went again to the funeral home to make the final payment and also travelled around town to make plans for the Repass. Colette was responsible for ordering food from a Chinese restaurant in Diego Martin and we chose the menu. We also rented table cloths from a catering service near the funeral home. The Repass was to take place at the parish hall of the church, and they provided tables and chairs. Colette said she would take care of the Repass and I could take care of the funeral program.

By afternoon, all arrangements were done and bills were paid. We then had time to pause. Saturday was going to be a free day. We decided to give ourselves the Saturday evening off for relaxation after a harrowing week and go to the Bishops Old Girls Carnival party. For the first time, I was actually in Trinidad for this event and took advantage of the opportunity. The party was bitter sweet experience because at the back of our heads was the impending funeral and no amount of music and merriment could drown that out.

Music of the Angels

The music director managed to get ten committed singers from the university choir to perform Fauré's Requiem. I asked him to suggest a fee for each student and was excited to have a rehearsal planned on the Sunday afternoon before the funeral. Two friends responded to my call for singers on Facebook and my friend Michelle, agreed to play the organ accompaniment. Things were looking promising.

I hadn't seen the music director since childhood when we participated in National Music Festival. I couldn't remember ever speaking to him back in the day, because I was too shy. However, he knew my name and face from participating in competitions in the past, and was delighted to help me. I was slightly amused when he asked who would conduct the Fauré. This was one dimension of the program I had never even considered. I knew I was delivering a eulogy and I was also singing for Mammy, but no thought was given as to who would lead the choir.

'I'm conducting the singers,' I said confidently, and then worried about adding another responsibility to my plate.

I hadn't conducted a choir in a long time. However, having sung in choirs for decades, I knew what to do. I felt conducting and running the program would also provide some distraction, so I wouldn't have to cry and feel sorry for myself through the whole service. Losing a mother who was solid as a rock was a big loss, and some distraction was needed.

The choir consisted of two sopranos, three altos, three tenors and three baritones. Because there were so few sopranos, I would also have to sing the soprano line and keep the melody going. This was an extra pressure.

We went through the music with the accompanist and the rehearsal was acceptable considering it was a last minute attempt. Everyone was asked to arrive at the church and hour in advance on Monday morning so we could warm up the voices and be ready to sing. One bass didn't show up for rehearsal and my voice was cracking during the rehearsal of my solo, the *Pie Jesu*. I decided to perform in a lower key on Monday morning because there was a strong possibility I would cry during the song and crack.

Tiffany and Amiri Arrive

My friend Joyanne offered to have Tiffany and me sleep at
her house Sunday night and take us directly to the church in
the morning. That was to relieve Brent of the responsibility
of getting everyone to the church on Monday morning on
time.

Tiffany was taking an international flight alone for the first
time, and I was a little apprehensive. I sent her an email
message with step by step instructions on all the documents
she needed, and reminders for changing planes in Miami.
Luckily her cousin, Amiri was also in transit from
Washington D.C. in Miami. They were scheduled to board
the same flight and would have each other for company. It
was an expensive ticket for just one day, flying out Tuesday
on the same flight as me. However, she came to pay her last
respects for the grandmother who took care of her when I
needed some time to finish my Ph.D. and also move to
California. It was the last goodbye.

Joyanne and her husband took me to meet Tiffany and Amiri
at the airport. We then settled Amiri at Brent's home and
were whisked away with our bags to Joyanne's place. I tried
to pack all the necessary items for the program and the
funeral in advance, and made many lists, checking them
twice and three times.

That night, I could barely sleep because of all the excitement
and anticipation of the funeral next day. I couldn't wait for it
to be over. I hoped the timing of the readings would be
right, the choir and organist would perform their entries on
time, and the priest would have patience with our lengthy
Requiem which replaced the typical choir hymns. I wanted
the program to be a musical triumph fit for Queen Mother
Gloria. For decades, she was a music teacher to many
students in our neighbourhood, as well as a music teacher at
Tranquillity Government Secondary School. She deserved it.

The Funeral Mass

The morning of the funeral, we heard on the news that a state funeral was also being held for the former President of Trinidad and Tobago. This meant certain road closures downtown and traffic everywhere. Luckily for Tiffany and me, we stayed in Cascade with Joyanne's family so it was an easy ride for us to arrive at the church an hour before the service was scheduled to start. I was worried though that some singers coming from the south of Trinidad and the organist coming from the east would be stuck in traffic. I called the organist on her cell phone and she complained of traffic with no end in site. At that stage, I considered plan B, which was to sing without accompaniment. It was time to pray.

St. Michael's and All Angels Anglican Church on the Wendy Fitzwilliams Boulevard in Diego Martin or 'Father Grey's Church' as we used to call it in childhood was the same church where our father's funeral was held. The building seemed to be timeless, appearing the same as in childhood.

When we arrived at the church, a neatly dressed, tall woman was observed fixing the altar, and fussing with setting up the podium for readings. I approached her to see if Tiffany could practise her reading since she hadn't done so before. She informed us the priest would get there shortly before the service started and I should give him a copy of the program.

Colette who was staying nearby in Diamond Vale arrived shortly after we got there. She arrived with flair wearing a black lace-lined dress with matching black fascinator neatly perched on top her neatly pulled back hair with long ponytail. A black scarf with silver floral print was draped over her shoulders for added decoration.

Soon after we arrived, the hearse pulled up with Mammy's coffin. The driver was a rotund, East Indian man with a small bald patch. He was dressed in a black shirt jacket and black trousers, which was probably the typical uniform from his company. As soon as he parked in front of the church, he retrieved a large container of food and started eating. This man must have risen early that morning and 8:00 am was as good a time as any to have a big meal. He ate what looked like rice and curried vegetables. After filling himself completely, he drank a bottle of cold water.

One hour before start time, the driver wheeled the coffin out to the front hall of the church. He had all the programs printed by the funeral home and we put them out on a table in the front of the church for people to take. I saved a few for choir members to follow as we sang. Colette asked the driver to open the coffin so we could see Mammy in her dress. She looked gaunt and ashy in her peach dress. We didn't stare for long and decided we would keep the casket closed, placing her framed black and white portrait on top. We wanted people to remember her former beauty.

I walked around wringing my hands nervously. I wondered when the singers would show up, if Brent and his family would arrive on time with the traffic, and if my Aunt Audrey and Kenrick would make it on time for the funeral. Brent had offered to collect my aunt and her husband but they said they would get someone to bring them. Well, close to the start of service they were not around and there was no telling if they would get to the funeral service.

When the priest arrived, I asked the church attendant to speak with him about the order of service. The priest was younger than I expected. Maybe I reminisced about the elderly priests from my childhood. Or maybe I was middle aged and those who I thought were elderly in my childhood may have been simply young adults and older than me. The priest sported a neatly cut afro and a confident air about him. When I gave him a copy of the program, he looked at it disapprovingly.

'Why didn't you send me a copy of the program to review?' he asked.

'Well, I sent a copy to what I thought was a church email address on Sunday. Perhaps I had the wrong address,' I replied.

I had to explain the Latin titles of movements from Fauré's Requiem and where I had placed them in the mass with communion. I thought all priests knew Latin because I didn't know where the *Pie Jesu* should fit. We agreed hastily on a revised order of service and I rushed out to let the choir know. In hind sight we should have asked for a simple lay service. The organist was not yet there so I decided to give her cues when it was time to play, based on the revised program.

Old neighbours and cousins walked into the church, so I went to the front to say a few hellos, and then walked back to the choir. My head was spinning. People I hadn't seen in years were filing in. At the eleventh hour, the organist arrived. She observed that the church organ was similar to hers and there was no need to bring her electric keyboard from the car. This was a welcome relief, because we had to start right away.

The Service

The priest entered in silence followed by the lay woman. Unfortunately I never thought of preparing an entrant hymn or organ interlude for the beginning of the funeral. The priest indicated that my siblings and I should read our eulogies at the beginning of the service since it was not part of a formal mass. Mine was filled with jokes about Mammy and the things she did in the past. I wondered if this speech was a bit raucous for church, but it was too late. Mammy liked to give jokes and wouldn't want a sombre funeral mass. Colette's and Brent's eulogies were short and to the point and then the singing started. The congregation may have been a little surprised by not being asked to sing the usual funeral dirges, but I wanted beautiful music fit for an angel. Our mother was an angel to us.

When the time came to sing my solo, the *Pie Jesu*, I tried not to cry. I focused on the notes and looked to the main entrance of the church. Luckily I started four tones lower and sang a cappella so everything went fine. Audrey and Kenrick walked in late and a little disoriented. I felt so sorry for them. They should have accepted our offer to stay overnight at Brent's home and arrive with the family. Marcus and Tiffany did excellent scriptural readings. When Amiri's turn came to read his passage, he started crying and wanted to read a speech he had written about his Granny. The service was already running late and there was no time for an adlib. We asked him to just read the Biblical passage and leave the podium, but he resisted for a few seconds which seemed like an eternity.

'But ... but ... I wrote a speech,' he protested.

'Just do the reading,' Brent and I urged him along.

Colette said nothing and hung her head down. She must have been thinking he was going to cause a stir as he had done on other occasions. Eventually he read the designated passage from the bible on the podium, and I motioned for him to sit with me so I could give him a hug. He burst into tears. Poor Amiri... Mammy had taken care of him for three years; from babe in arms to his toddler years and he missed her dearly. In addition, Colette had not spoken to him in months and this deepened the loss of his grandmother.

After the last movement, *In Paridisum*, I rushed to pay the choir and thanked them. I had prepared hand written cards with payment for the names of ten students and also thank you cards for two friends who sang with us. To my shock, an additional student sang with us that morning. Luckily I had brought extra cash in my purse just in case of an emergency. As the leader of the choir approached me for their fees, I gave him the stack of neatly written cards then ask him to give the extra student the cash in hand.

With profuse thanks I then rushed to the main entrance of the church to greet guests who were leaving. Even though the program mentioned the Repass in the Parish Hall, I still wanted to remind people to wait around. We still had to drive to Lapeyrouse Cemetery in Woodbrook, some 15 kilometres away, for the burial. Then we planned to drive back to the Parish Hall in Diego Martin. It was going to be a small feat to squeeze in everything smoothly.

'Oh Auntie Cynthia, and is that Corinne? I haven't seen you all in decades!'

I saw school friends, neighbours, cousins, and some vaguely familiar faces that looked decades older than their former selves. I was embarrassed not to recognise so many people and remember their names. During the meet and greet, my aunt Audrey fell to the ground. With all the excitement, she was probably dehydrated and sick. After all, she was diabetic and suffering from dementia, so nobody knew what happened. The last thing we needed was another casualty in the family. Luckily two retired nurses were present, and someone brought her a chair as they tried to revive her with water.

During the incident, the pall bearers had wheeled Mammy's coffin to the hearse. Before I knew it, the driver took off at full speed to Lapeyrouse Cemetery. I thought he would wait to have a procession of cars to the burial ground. Maybe that was a thing of the past. We certainly never thought to give him instructions before the funeral, so he did what he wanted. Joyanne had volunteered to take me around that day, so I managed to seek her out and we left for the cemetery immediately.

Thankfully, roads were quiet in the middle of the day and we arrived at the cemetery in record time. The grave diggers were waiting at the site and a slight drizzle began to fall. We saw the red dirt flung in a big mound at the side of a plot with the tombstone engraved, 'In Memory of Joey Braithwaite'. It was then it hit me why we couldn't' find the tombstone the previous week. We were looking for one with the family name, Irish, since my grandparents were Stella and Rupert Irish, and my aunt Pearl Irish were buried there. In fact, Aunt Pearl who was adopted by the Braithwaite family inherited this plot and then left it in her Will for us.

As we gathered around the burial site, some of our former neighbours from Diamond Vale started singing the typical funeral dirges which I found so mournful. I burst into tears immediately after holding up very well for the past few days. Amiri was able to read a well written tribute to his grandmother at the grave site before the staff lowered her body into the hole. That part was the most difficult for me. Hearing the gravel hit the casket, sealing her body in a box seemed like a horrible ending for anyone, especially Mammy.

Aunt Betty uttered the same sentiment, 'They say that she's in a better place. Well if that's what you call a better place, I don't want it!'

I burst into tears again. I had to cry out all the pent up emotions from days, weeks, months, and years of being strong. There was nothing left but to release as much as possible through sobbing. When I was able to compose myself, we took photos at the graveside and I felt relieved. I promised myself to return one day to put a new tombstone on the grave, writing all the names of family buried there. The name of my beloved mother had to be etched in stone.

The Repass

We left the burial ground to return to the parish hall for a celebration of Mammy's life.

The Parish Hall situated right next to the church was a concrete block building painted pastel yellow with a large polished, cement terrazzo floor. The open structure mirrored that of the church for good air circulation. Restrooms were situated on the western side of the building. A stage and storage room for tables and chairs were on the eastern side. Towards the back of the building was a kitchen space equipped with sinks, and a counter ideal for serving food and drinks. The church supplied six foot tables and red chairs which fit well with the white table cloths to dress the tables.

It had been a long morning and everyone was hungry. Colette reminded me that since I took charge of the funeral service, she was going to be in charge of the Repass. I said OK, but somehow could never help myself in taking over event planning. I let her take care of the food. She had enlisted the help of her friends to dress the tables and serve drinks while we went to the burial ground. Joyanne's brother was responsible for setting up music and playing during the service. Kim's daughter prepared a creative slide show of Mammy's life, using photos that I'd sent her. We borrowed a slide projector and I set the slide show in motion with my laptop, so people could look at this while they sat at the tables.

I suggested that people serve themselves. The caterer had

delivered the food before we returned from the cemetery and I felt we'd ordered too much. Many people had left after the funeral service to return to work or home, and didn't stay around for lunch. Colette said she wanted to serve people and that was final. Well, I tried staying out of the way focused on getting my own lunch. When most people had eaten, I borrowed the DJs microphone and started telling stories and jokes about Mammy's life. After all, it was supposed to be a celebration and she always liked to tell stories. I invited her old friend Petra to the say a few words on the microphone and we got a short glimpse of their relationship. Mammy's friend Kim couldn't speak and only cried when she tried to tell a few tales. Others were a little shy, and Colette and Brent may have been too exhausted after the past few days. Amiri told an off-colour joke and I took the microphone away from him, before he went too far in the wrong direction.

The party was filled with cousins from my dad side who also loved Mammy. She was one of the last survivors from that era and everyone came out to support. This was heart warming to see. As the party wrapped up, we had mountains of food left over for people to take away. It was a day well spent and we were all relieved it went well.

Travelling Back

The next drama was flying out of Trinidad. I felt that Brent and his family had endured enough excitement with all the visitors, and would be thankful when we returned to our respective homes, so they could have peace and quite again. Amiri checked online and observed that his connecting flight from Houston to Washington D.C. was cancelled because of a snow storm. He wanted to spend more days in Trinidad. We all pushed him to get on his way and find an alternate route to his final destination home. I told him his Uncle

Brent had too many visitors and we had to leave and give him some time with family. Brent took him to the airport that night with a bit of fretting and confusion. Fortunately a deal was worked out at the airline counter and he was able to leave.

On Tuesday 16th January, Colette, Tiffany and I woke up at 4:30 am to catch our early morning flights back to Florida and Canada respectively. Every bone in my body ached. My brain felt tired from the whole experience of Mammy's death and the planning of the funeral. I wasn't sure how I was going to recover from that week, but felt satisfied we had organised the best farewell we could for our dear mother.

Gloria James is making music with the angels in heaven.

May she rest in Peace.

## WHO WAS GLORIA JAMES?

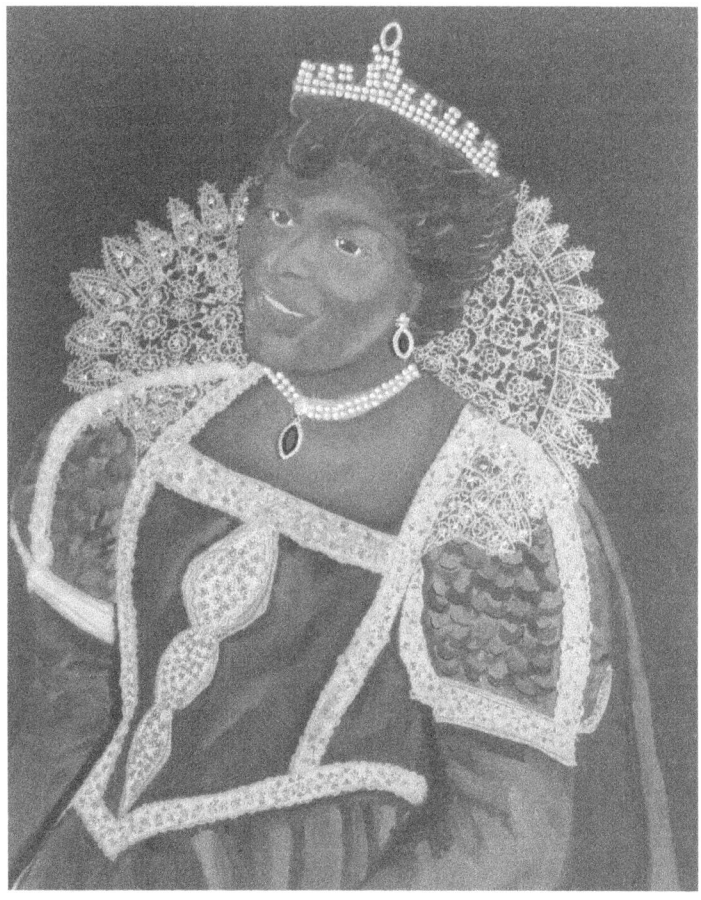

'Queen Mother Glory', acrylic on canvas, 24"x30", painted by Jennylynd James.
https://jennylyndjames.pixels.com/

Mammy, Gloria James, born Gloria Eileen Irish on December 29th, 1932 was raised in Belmont, Port-of-Spain, Trinidad and Tobago. She was the second child and eldest daughter of Stella and Rupert Irish and had three brothers: Wallace,

Ponceford and Edgar, and two sisters: Pearl and Audrey.

Mammy was a tomboy and by all accounts, her father's favourite child. She attended St Margaret's Girls' Anglican School (also called Melville Memorial). She then attended Osmond High School (or Murray School), where she sat the Senior Cambridge School Certificate Examinations passing five subjects. After leaving school, career choices seemed limited, and she decided to study typing and short hand to become a secretary. Later on, she discovered a love for teaching and enrolled as a student teacher. Her first assignment was at Manzanilla Government Primary School.

She told us fond stories about the beautiful country people of Manzanilla who gathered every Sunday evening to greet Teacher Gloria as she arrived in the one and only taxi running between Sangre Grande and Manzanilla. She boarded with a family in Manzanilla, returning to her city home in Belmont on Friday evenings.

Mammy attended the Teacher's Training College where she met my father, Kenneth James. They got married after graduation on August 11th, 1962. She taught for 34 years in the public school system. This included Mount D'Or Government, San Juan Government, Eastern Boys Government Primary School, and finally at Tranquility Government Secondary School, where she retired as a Music Teacher. Mammy also gave piano lessons at our home in Diamond Vale.

GLO-RI-AH, as I liked to call her, enjoyed preparing students for piano exams and school choirs for the Trinidad and Tobago National Music Festival. She was a member of the Music Teacher's Association and served as President of the Senior Achievers Association of Retired Persons.

Mammy introduced me to music at a young age and

cultivated in me a love of music. When I was five years old she started teaching me to play the piano and I continued for years, entering competitions in the National Music Festival and taking exams. Even though I was shy, she gently encouraged me to play on the 12 and under show on TV, and to also work as an accompanist at a ballet school. Solo performances and choir participation were thrust upon me and she provided every possible support. To this day, I still sing and participate in musical events and greatly appreciate all the musical training I received in Trinidad.

Mammy taught me about saving and investing. She would always say, 'No matter how much money you make, always put aside some for a rainy day'. She was brilliant at investing and budgeting, and was eager to pass on her knowledge. After graduating from high school, I worked for a year to 'learn the value of money' as my father would say, before leaving home to study in Canada. Mammy made sure I invested some of my earnings that year by taking me to a stock broker's office to buy some stocks in a local company poised for growth. She taught me about government bonds and term savings accounts. Anything she had learned from others about investing, she taught me and I absorbed it like a sponge.

Time management was one of her strengths. Living in Diego Martin and working in Port-of-Spain had its challenges with traffic, even back in the late 70's. Mammy would wake up at 5 am, cook lunch, and pack meals for everyone to take to school or work. We would eat breakfast as a family and then leave for Port-of-Spain by 6:15 am to avoid traffic. Timing was everything. After working as a teacher at a school in Port-of-Spain, she gave piano lessons at home and then sometimes helped us with homework. She worked tirelessly for everyone and I wonder if she even had a minute for herself.

Mammy always wanted to help those less fortunate than us.

As children, we were asked to collect our unwanted toys and books at Christmastime to give to others. Everyone who passed the house asking for help got some form of charity if they helped us too; for example, cleaning the garden or doing small chores. Christmastime was also special because Mammy prepared a package or a case of beers for the postman, the garbage man and others who served the community all year long.

Mammy loved to gather people together for entertainment and parties. Every year, just after Christmas, we would have a dinner party and invite everyone we knew to the house. Most of the time, the event coincided with her birthday. Cleaning, decorating, and cooking up a storm for the party were a joy for us … never a chore.

Mammy had said, 'Feeding many people at home brings good luck and riches', and I still believe it to this today.

Mammy was strict, but loving and kind as she moulded many aspects of our lives childhood well into adulthood. I am eternally grateful to her for helping to care for my daughter, Tiffany, at a time when I had to finish my Ph.D. and also when I relocated to California. Her generous spirit paved the path for my success today and I will miss her more than words can say.

I love you GLO-RI-AH.

## VICTIM STATEMENT - THE END IS NEAR

I'm lying on a single bed

I'm skinnier than I've ever been in my whole life

The room is dark and an old woman is in a single bed on the other side of the room

She is not moving or speaking, but her eyes are open wide, staring at the ceiling

They put me on my side and my right leg is bent … can't straighten it out

Why can't I straighten this leg out?

I can't feel my feet

Getting cramps in my bony hip

Staring at the wall, I can see the sun peeping through the window

'Gloria time to eat your lunch'

The girl has a kind soft voice

She forces me to sit up and I scream in pain.

It's so painful to move in any direction

I try to hit her … think I will bite her when she tries to move me again

Ha … I got her …

'Ouch', she yells …

She props me to sit up and feeds me one spoonful of soup at

a time …

It tastes good. I think … What is this soup she is feeding me?

Why can't I hold the spoon? I move my hands but she tells me to wait. She feeds me

Wait … I am still hungry, but I can't eat … So hungry …

Did I get anything to eat?

Commotion outside

'Your friends are here for your birthday,' the girl said.

'We have to dress you'.

I close my eyes. They can't seem to open … I feel so weak

The girl puts me to lie down and takes off the pee soaked pamper

She wipes me and puts on a new one

My body is exposed … The indignity … The shame …

My legs are exposed. My bottom is exposed for all to see

The old woman is lying on the bed on the other side of the room motionless, staring at the ceiling

I scream out in pain

She says 'Be quiet'; what does that mean?

I am in pain when the nice girl moves my legs to wipe my bottom.

She puts on a new pamper and takes off my dirty nightgown

'This is a pretty dress,' she says.

'Your friends are here for your birthday'

My eyes are closed. What dress did she put on me?

She lifts me up and I land bottom first on the seat of a wheelchair

I scream as body hits the hard leather seat. Oh the pain...

'We're going out now,' she says

I grab onto the arms of the wheelchair. The motion frightens me...

I can't move my legs...

We are in another room

'Hello Gloria! Happy birthday!'

I can't open my eyes... my head feels so heavy... Why I can't I open my eyes? Who are these people?

My body is numb

'Eat some cake! Happy birthday to you! Happy birthday to you!'

Why are they singing this? How old am I? Who are these people?

My body aches all over. The pain!

Eventually they leave and the nice girl rolls me back in the wheelchair

The world is spinning

Can't open my eyes

I can't breathe.

'Something is wrong. Come and see her,' said the girl

The man asked the girl to take me to the emergency ward

Someone wheels me to a car. I'm so afraid. I sit in a seat and we are moving somewhere. My eyes are closed and I'm so weak.

Can't breathe … can't breathe

We are in a noisy room. They put me on a hard bed... Ouch!

Noise and people… noise and people…

Who are all these people running, running all the time?

They stick me with needles and I can't see.

'I have to go home now,' said the nice girl. 'You'll be alright.'

I'm so cold. I don't know anybody. So hungry, no food … no food

They stick me with another needle.

Ouch! Ouch! They are hurting me

'Let's do a CAT scan and some blood work'

They put a hard plastic mask over my nose.

Now I can breathe… Oh now I can breathe…

It's so cold. So many people, up and down

Where am I? Why is it so noisy?

Who are these strangers? Is it day? Is it night?

How long have I been here? Noise, noise, noise...

'Discharge her and send her home,' said one voice. 'She's an old woman. We can't do much for her and we need the bed.'

The bed is rolling. They take off the mask from my nose. I try to breathe.

They put me somewhere. I can't open my eyes.

Some men said they have to drive up that big hill. The road is too steep

The nice girl puts me in the wheelchair again and I'm now on the single bed again

'Gloria eat some soup,' she said.

I'm hungry, but I don't want it.

One day, two days, three days ... I'm hungry, but I cannot eat.

My head is spinning. I can't feel my body

An electric jolt hit me.

'Oh my God, Gloria is on the ground!'

Noise and commotion

'Let's take her to the Emergency Ward right away. We don't have any equipment here. She can't even breathe.'

I can't feel my arms and legs. My eyes are closed. I can feel the motion. We are driving somewhere.

The same noise like before. People running, running, screaming people. Needles in both arms

'Trying to get her pulse. Give her oxygen. She can't stay here. Put her in the adult ward.'

More needles in my arms. I'm so cold. So hungry.

Where am I? Who are these people?

So cold, so hungry, so alone

The world is spinning.

'She's an old woman. She will die soon.'

They put me on a bed, two arms outstretched and head to one side.

My body is placed on the side. I can't bend the right leg.

They cover me with a cloth. I can't move my head, my arms, and my legs

Cramps in my arms... Can't move them. Nobody moves them.

Other people are in the room. I know they are. I can't see them.

People come and go.

They check my arm. Nobody speaks to me.

Some people talk about me. 'She's an old woman. Not good. She'll probably die soon.'

I can hear them

I can't move my head. The hard plastic mask over my nose is digging into my right eye. Can somebody move this? They haven't seen this.

It's painful. I can't speak

The room is quiet.

She comes to visit. 'Mammy, I'm your daughter. I came to see you. Are you OK?'

She holds my hand and cries. Who is my daughter?

More people come to visit and look at me. I can't open my eyes. I can feel their presence.

A large group is there.

'Gloria, everyone came to see you. Lindy, Colette, Brent, Audrey, Kenrick'

They talk loudly at my bedside.

It's too much noise… They are so loud. He pinches my toe.

Ouch… I move my leg. I can feel my foot …

So much pain. My body is heavy and cold.

I can't hold on … They are all looking at me.

The next day the doctor speaks to all of them.

I can hear them

'We recommend Palliative Care. She'll never get better.

Give permission for no resuscitation. She could die any day …'

What does this mean? Is it time to give up?

I'm hungry. The pamper is dirty. I cannot move.

My head is lying on one side, my two arms spread out

Some familiar voices are arguing.

'At least they could have changed her. They didn't feed her by syringe.

The food is still sitting there. She has bed sores.

Oh my God they are wicked here.

The oxygen mask is digging into her eye. Fix it!

She's been in the same position for the two days since I've been here.

Move her body to the other side!'

Noise! Shouting!

Two people clean me. I'm lying on the next side.

I still can't breathe.

Can't open my eyes. Who are all these people?

They hug me and say goodbye.

They all leave me alone. I know they love me.

I WANT TO DIE

I AM TIRED

Can't breathe … drifting … no more pain …


THE END

Jennylynd James

# ABOUT THE AUTHOR

Jennylynd James is a "Renaissance" woman: an artist, writer, and musician with a long work history as a food scientist. Jennylynd earned a Ph.D. in Food Science at McGill University, Canada and worked in this field for over 20 years for large multinational companies in the United States, Ireland, and Canada. While living in Ireland she ran her own food processing business. When the Irish economy crashed on the heels of a worldwide recession, Jennylynd decided to fold up the business and move to Canada. Jennylynd lives in Toronto, Canada where she has embraced self expression in art, music, and writing as a new lifestyle. Jennylynd has written a series of travel memoirs to chronicle her many adventures in relocation. 'Where are my Car Keys?' describes her mother's slow demise with Alzheimer's disease from 2006 to 2018. Jennylynd, with her daughter, Tiffany work through the challenges of relocation, while making numerous visits to Trinidad and Tobago to visit her ailing mother. She hopes to touch the reader by evoking an understanding of all the emotions involved in living in a foreign country, while her parents age, become ill, and eventually die. She wants her stories of resilience and thriving to empower and motivate readers.

http://jennylyndjames.com/books